EXECUTIVE EASE AND DIS-EASE

For

Sir Richard Powell Bt. MC

whose foresight and support
made all this work possible

EXECUTIVE EASE AND DIS-EASE

H. Beric Wright MB, FRCS

Medical Adviser Institute of Directors
Chief Medical Officer BUPA Ltd.

A HALSTED PRESS BOOK

JOHN WILEY & SONS
New York – Toronto

First published in Great Britain by Gower Press Limited, Epping, Essex
1975

© H. Beric Wright 1975

Published in the U.S.A.
by Halsted Press, a Division
of John Wiley & Sons, Inc.
New York

Library of Congress Cataloging in Publication Data

Wright, Henry Beric.
  Executive ease and dis-ease.
  "A Halsted Press book."
  1. Executives—Health programs. 2. Hygiene.
3. Stress (Psychology) I. Title.
RA776.5.W74 1975   613'.02'4658   75-1072
ISBN 0-470-96450-2

Printed & bound in Great Britain

Contents

Illustrations

Acknowledgments

Dr Guido Pincherle, who was then Head of the Medical Research Department at the Institute of Directors, and I started to write this book in 1968/9. We hoped to get it finished before we moved The Medical Centre in the spring of 1970. Unfortunately, the pressure of life and the problems of learning how to be married to a computer, did not permit any serious writing time until recently. By then Dr Pincherle had joined the Department of Health and Social Security so I had to press on alone. However, I would like to express my appreciation of all he did as our first full-time research worker to point The Medical Centre's research activity in the right general direction, and to thank him for his personal support.

Although the ideas presented here represent my own views and experience, they have evolved from the common experience that we have had together at The Medical Centre over the past ten years and I would not expect all my medical colleagues to agree with everything I have said. However, I would like to thank them particularly, those who joined us in the early years, for their help and support. We are now an accepted part of the country's medical life, but in the early days one needed a small dash of martyrdom to work as a doctor for the Institute of Directors. We have, I hope, developed our ideas on environmental medicine as a team sailing into what was originally uncharted water. Although the crew were sometimes mutinous, I appreciate their joining the team.

The Governors of BUPA Medical Centre Ltd, representing BUPA and the Institute of Directors, were good enough to let me have two months' leave of absence during which I finally wrote the book. I very much appreciate their willingness to do this and can only hope, for their sakes, that any possible precedent created by this absence will not be embarrassing.

Without the detailed and boring work undertaken by my own staff, the book could never have been put together. Dr Alan Bailey, now Head of Research, and Mr David Robinson, our Statistician, were good enough to produce the tables and figures while Mrs Carolyn Kent provided typing and compilation with unfailing good will and skill. To all of them, and my family, my heartfelt thanks and gratitude.

Lastly, I must congratulate the publishers on their persistent patience, courtesy and finally speed.

H. Beric Wright
Quainton, Bucks

Introduction

Health and effectiveness

Does health matter?

Ask any manager which aspect of his work or area of responsibility causes him the most worry or anxiety and nine out of ten will reply: 'people'. Plant, capital, premises and ideas, manufacturing, storing, distribution, marketing and selling, all involve people. The main task of the senior manager should be to create an environment in which people — individual people — can flourish to the mutual benefit of themselves and the enterprise. In order to flourish his staff or colleagues must be reasonably fit and well. In popular terms they should be 'healthy'.

As we shall see in the course of this book, being healthy involves mental as well as physical factors. Health is difficult to define because it covers so many aspects of the individual's relationship with his environment. The World Health Authority, shortly after the war, defined health as 'a state of mental, physical and social well-being'. This definition recognized officially, perhaps for the first time, that health was likely to involve more than the mere absence of disease. It could be, for instance, that the way in which one lived and worked might play a major part in determining whether or not one was 'ill'. Certainly, we in The Medical Centre* believe this to be true and it is a

---

* The Medical Centre in London, as well as offering businessmen a specialized service, operates the largest computerized health check unit in Europe. It is run by BUPA (British United Provident Association) with Institute of Directors representation on the Board of Directors.

concept which conditions all our thinking about the problems of executive health.

With the techniques presently available to experimental medicine, or the behavioural sciences, it is almost impossible to demonstrate either a relationship between general fitness and executive effectiveness or to measure health. Although obviously at the extremes of the spectrum of performance, someone who is unconscious because of a diabetic or alcoholic coma is unlikely to be able to take decisions, but equally, an invalid or someone with heart failure, can often think effectively for short periods.

In general terms, however, the proposition that fit, well people are likely to be more effective and efficient must rest on common sense. Although there is a little experimental evidence to suggest that a reasonable degree of physical fitness is conducive to more sustained and effective mental effort, at any rate for average people, it also probably adds a reserve of resilience to deal with the extra demand of crises.

If then management involves people, and health is related to effectiveness, senior managers must be concerned about health — their own and that of the people for whom they are responsible and on whose motivation and skills they are dependent. It is also worth making the point that people may be a company's least replaceable asset. In small or medium sized organizations particularly, the loss of one key person for whom there is no trained deputy can be devastating if not disastrous. If, too, the owner of a small company is incapacitated, the livelihood of all his workers as well as his family is at stake. He owes it to both of them to look after himself sensibly.

The Medical Centre believes that the responsibility for maintaining health should be a reflection of the basic relationship between the individual and the organization for which he works, ie the responsibility is mutual; it is in the best interests of both parties that reasonable steps are taken to live and work sensibly and not too demandingly.

There is, however, a type of person, usually domineering and self-centred, who often seems determined to drive himself to destruction. Nothing a doctor, wife or colleague can say or recommend appears to make much difference to this man's way of life. If he is lucky he may get a mild coronary which frightens him back to a more sensible existence. If he is unlucky he dies in some foreign hotel and leaves a widow, two children under fourteen, and a rather miserable pension, to say nothing of a gaping hole within the organization.

As will be shown, coronary thrombosis is the biggest single killer of middle-aged men. Many of the factors which contribute to coronary proneness are related to the individual's way of life and thus largely under his control.

Coronary proneness can to a degree be predicted by medical examination and advice to modify one's way of life or the treatment of predisposing factors, like early increased blood pressure (hypertension) or raised cholesterol, can now often minimize the chances of getting a heart attack. For these and many other reasons there is a relationship between the health of the individual and the success of the enterprise with which he is associated. To this extent at least, executive health and its maintenance is a topic not without importance. To be concerned about it is a reflection of prudence rather than hypochondria.

General medical experience also lends some support to arguments in favour of the value of preventive maintenance on people. After all, if one services plant, machinery and motor cars, why not look at individuals in the same way, before rather than after they break down?

A relatively large number of screening surveys have been carried out in various countries, on population groups of different ages and socio-economic status. All of them, including a number in this country, have revealed what has come to be called 'the hidden iceberg of disease'. Disease which has caused measurable or detectable changes in one or more body systems without necessarily producing symptoms sufficient to drive the individual to his doctor.

In this respect it is also worth noting that many reasonably robust and well-adjusted people put up with a wide range of symptoms and disabilities, the alleviation or mitigation of which is both possible and likely to make their lives easier or more comfortable. The busier and more involved a person is, the more important it is that he does not waste energy and effort overcoming even the simplest medical disabilities.

Unfortunately, executive life is physically relatively undemanding; if one can stagger out of the car, across the hall into the lift and out as far as the office, one is 'in business' and can work. A physically more demanding job might lead to a higher standard of health and fitness, if only to make it possible to hold down the job.

There is no doubt that some members of the 'tycoon class' do suffer from the 'it can't happen to me' syndrome, with consequent reduction of their life expectancy.

That there is a potential iceberg of disease in executives is borne out by some of the figures from the experience of The Medical Centre over the last ten years (see Chapters 2 and 3). In general terms, and as a result of many thousands of executive health examinations, it can be said that about 30 per cent of those seen have actual or potential disease which is worth dealing with. This is as true for the young as it is for the old.

There is also a similar, if less easy to detect iceberg, of what now can be reasonably and respectably called 'mental ill-health'. This does not only mean overt mental breakdown leading to hospitalization and dramatic treatment like electric shock or leucotomy (disconnecting one part of the brain by cutting the connections with a knife) but also the much more common frustration, anxiety, insomnia, dyspepsia, depression, declining libido and general lack of enjoyment or satisfaction out of life, which is not nowadays all that uncommon in middle-aged business men.

Stress symptoms of this type contribute to poor health and loss of efficiency; they often arise from a bad balance between the individual and his environment (work, home and leisure). Dealing with this situation may involve altering the environment, a change of job, more or less responsibility, a holiday, a divorce, a new boss, all of which factors can play a part in determining health.

It is not yet really possible to measure the parameters of health any more than the individual items which contribute to management effectiveness can be seriously pinpointed. Health, like efficiency and effectiveness, is compounded of elusive, complicated and somewhat subjective qualities. But under the various headings so far outlined it is hoped that the reader will agree that there are good grounds for believing that not only does the executive's health matter, but also that it is an area in which given reasonable cooperation by the individual, his wife and his work, an increasing amount can be done to avoid the pitfalls and minimize the chances of medical disaster. This is really what this book is about.

How demanding is management?

In discussing the importance of executive health and the perhaps privileged facilities that are available to advise about it, it is difficult not to get embroiled in semi-philosophical arguments of the type: 'no one group of people can be regarded as more important than another', or 'only the wealthy or the subsidized can afford *that* sort of advice'.

Up to the time that the Institute of Directors started to take an interest in the occupational health problems of the businessman, it was, I think, justified to say that he took considerably less interest in his own problems than he did in those of the rest of his staff. Most large manufacturing firms, for instance, had medical departments, but they were primarily for the shop-floor worker. We were able to point out, for the kind of reasons already outlined, that the executive group did, in fact, have medical problems which could be and needed to be dealt with. In addition, there were grounds for believing that the sedentary, cigarette smoking, managerial and professional group in this country appeared to have a higher coronary thrombosis rate than other socio-economic groups.

Against this background, it can be said that key people who may be 'at risk' — in just the same way as the man exposed to toxic hazards — should also be similarly medically monitored. Managers have the responsibility of taking decisions which can make or break the organization. They create wealth on which the survival of the community depends. They also create, not always for the best, the environment which the rest of the employees inhabit. The skills required to do this successfully are not easily acquired and are not all that widely distributed throughout the population. We believe that they are worth preserving.

There are also two political facets to this argument. The first involves the principle of withholding something seemingly desirable until such time as it can be made available to everyone. The second involves the preservation of centres of specialization or excellence. Both facets are now being applied to medicine and education and amount roughly to a decision as to whether the Government wants to try to level people upwards or downwards.

I have always hoped that health maintenance will become part of the health, rather than sickness, service, but until it so becomes, I am happy to continue to try to demonstrate its value by making it available to an important minority group who appear to want it and are prepared, increasingly, to buy it.

It may be said, particularly by those without experience, that decision taking is easy, rewarding and stimulating. The latter two it may be, but in this day and age it is seldom easy. There is no simple answer to complex problems and, particularly over the last ten years, the parameters or the ground rules on which decisions are taken change with bewildering speed.

A great number of conflicting interests have to be resolved: the shareholders, the bankers, the workers (individually and through their unions), local and central government and so on. To give one simple example: before World War II, it was not too difficult to buy a plot of land, deal with the local byelaws and put up a factory. Now, the chances are high that the factory will have to be built 200 miles from the existing manufacturing unit and shipyard workers or miners retrained to staff it.

Running a business successfully is largely a matter of forecasting demand, costs and profits. I well remember seeing the chairman of a large international company at the time the Labour government of 1966-70 announced the introduction of Corporation Tax, import surcharge and the cutting of overseas investments. Until the rates for some of these were announced in six months' time, no plans for the future could be made. Similarly, the sudden introduction of SET completely altered the costing of many business activities. Managers have to be tough to survive in this climate. Now the climate is getting harsher and the work less rewarding.

Since the war, it has been technologically possible to cram so much more into the managerial day or week than it was previously. Telephones, teleprinters, closed circuit television, computers and aeroplanes have measurably increased the pace of life. It is now both possible to, and expected that one should, do more in the day than even ten years ago. Before the war, for instance, it was virtually impossible to get to America in less than five days.

Another factor here, particularly for the British manager, is that until recently he has not been given much technical training. Technology and business procedures, which have been developed since he left school, put an increasing strain on the middle-aged manager. He often left school at 15 or 16 and never kept on learning to learn. He then gets stressed because he finds it difficult to keep up and is frightened of being pushed aside by bright youngsters. This makes him prone to stress diseases. Management consultants and computers moving into a company provide just this sort of stress situation.

The manager's way of life, as determined by fashion and behaviour of his peers, is not conducive to longevity. Endless trivial meetings, travel at home and overseas, lunches, dinners, conferences and paper work done largely out of office hours, all add up to a long week and short weekend.

In the course of this book, I shall need to elaborate on many of these points, but I suggest that they make good grounds for believing that although the rewards and satisfactions are high, management is an extremely demanding activity. It can no longer be done by gifted amateurs by the seat of their pants. Good health has become an essential part of successful managerial survival.

What is health?

To understand the medical philosophy underlying the advice on living sensibly and within one's limitations, is the purpose of this book. It is thus necessary to look, in more detail, at our concept of health and the way in which it relates to illness and performance. Two basic points are, hopefully, already apparent. Firstly, that health is more than the mere absence of disease, and secondly, that it is a reflection of the way in which the individual deals with the environment. To understand the implications of this concept we need to know a little more about the way in which personality and behavioural factors influence what might loosely be called resistance or proneness to disease. The phrase 'disease' needs also to be qualified or divided into two groups of afflictions: the organic and the behavioural.

When I was a medical student, complaints for which no detectable physical change could be found were called functional and the patient written off as neurotic. It is now realized that the mental often determines the physical and that complaints or symptoms are a call for help from a distressed person. The fact that there is nothing to show for the symptoms is little measure of their reality to the sufferer. The probability is that diseases for which there is no effective cure, like rheumatoid arthritis, psoriasis or migraine, may have a large mental or psychological element. Perhaps when we can understand more about the processes involved, we shall be on the threshold of doing something about reversing them, rather than merely trying to suppress the symptoms with powerful and often dangerous drugs.

To give a less medically complicated example, it is relatively easy to control the symptoms of indigestion with alkalis, or even to ask a surgeon to remove a duodenal ulcer. But surgery apart, the chances of a real cure are reduced without understanding *why* the individual has these symptoms. What is it in the relationship between him and his environment that has produced this reaction?

One of the best illustrations of this concerns a salesman in a print business who, about a year previously, had undergone a large operation for gastric haemorrhage. This had been done at a well-known teaching hospital, but it had not cured his symptoms. He was becoming increasingly miserable in spite of having had a lot of time off work and being sent by the company, with his wife on a splendid cruise.

The man was by now about 50. His story, which was ellicited without difficulty, was as follows. He married at the outset of the war in a hurry and was away for several years doing quite well as a technical NCO. After a year or so, his wife left him, which was bad for his pride, but there was nothing he could do about it but divorce her. He was an only son and on demobilization he lived happily with his mother and did well at his job. Occasionally he went out with a girl; not much happened, but this did not worry him. Finally, about two years before I saw him, his mother died. Six months or so after this, his secretary, of many years association, dragged him slightly reluctantly to the altar. Having got him hooked, she was dismayed to find him impotent. The resulting conflict and anxiety produced a serious ulcer, but the surgery did nothing to deal with the cause, and rather bizarre and disconcerting symptoms continued.

This case history, described in some detail, illustrates the basis of psychosomatic or 'whole man' medicine. The experience goes back well over ten years, but the surgeon was very angry when I suggested that he might have got the full story before deciding to operate.

Our concept of disease has two implications which permeate the whole of our thinking. The first is that *why* a person is ill, ie why he has symptoms or shows changes, may be just as important as *what* is wrong with him or her. Indeed, in the proper understanding of the 'illness situation' it is often more important.

The second is that the diseases people get are often related to the lives they lead, and again to understand the illness one needs to know a great deal more than just its symptoms, what they are and when they started. One of the great difficulties here is that people, quite subconsciously, tend to make excuses to visit the doctor. Tradition can play a great part in the confrontation between doctor and patient and 'respectable' symptoms are presented, when the real trouble is quite different or more complicated, like sexual frigidity or anxiety about a child's behaviour. Similarly, a businessman with quite severe insomnia or dyspepsia may well not have had a holiday and be extremely worried about the difficulty of raising capital for the vital extension of his business, or be bothered by an ageing and perhaps related chairman whose business thinking comes from a previous generation.

This is known technically as the psychosomatic basis of disease. Psychosomatic broadly means mind (psyche) and body (soma). Disease is thus a reflection of the interrelationship between the mind and the body, or the mental and the physical. In these terms, it is unimportant which system reflects the disease; what is important is that an imbalance has occurred and the basic relationship has been upset. Of course, physical disease is still much more respectable than mental, but it is at last being realized by doctors and the public that the two are but opposite ends of the total spectrum of disturbed behaviour.

At long last, it is beginning to be possible to get people to accept that there is no inherent difference between an acute anxiety state and, say, pneumonia or appendicitis: both are medical emergencies involving hospitalization and urgent treatment. It has taken a long time to reach this stage in our thinking because up to recently there was so much infectious and other disease. Higher standards of living and effective drugs have reduced the incidence of this type of illness. Tuberculosis, pneumonia, rheumatic fever and even appendicitis seem much rarer. But in spite of all this, in spite of the health service, drugs, hospitals and the welfare state, the illness rate, as reflected in sickness absence figures, goes up rather than down.

Certified sickness as reflected in absenteeism and demand for sick pay, has gone steadily up over the last twenty years and is now at over 400 million days per year. This is a measure of the community's inability to deal with its problems rather than an index of overt illness. The certificates will say influenza, general malaise, debility, and so on, but they largely mean that the individual is unwilling to work and that the community accepts this by paying high benefits and not questioning the real need for the certificate.

All living things are in a constant state of reaction with their environment, to the pressures and demands of which they have to adjust. It is the challenge of having to make this adjustment that gives biological life its tone and provides the stimulus for evolution. Plants compete with each other for nutrition and with the general climatic environment for heat and moisture. Fishes, birds and animals similarly have to battle for food and to be able to survive the climate. The same used to be true for man: he too fought on two fronts, the environment and the interpersonal. As far as man is concerned, recent political problems apart, the physical environment now presents relatively little challenge. Provided the individual or the community can pay the bill, the house keeps out the elements; water, heat and light are available and food can be bought. The major source of friction or conflict for man is now from his fellow men.

Overcoming environmental challenge is the stimulus for existence and the spur of evolutionary change. The need for challenge is a basic requirement of life and provides its satisfaction. If this is so, as an equally basic feature of living things, there is likely to be a defence mechanism against too much challenge. At this stage in the argument there is no need to be anthropomorphic about the reactions of animals, except to note in passing that animals do get stress diseases and that the studies of Tinbergen and Lorenz have shown that 'herds' of birds, fishes and animals, leading a crowded existence, do develop both defence mechanisms and stress diseases, in response to the pressures of community life. They also develop the most fascinating behaviour patterns to control these conflicts. Man is on the whole the only species that 'preys' on his own kind.

The human animal then, must have a defence mechanism against too much challenge. He needs some respectable way of running away from, or opting out of, an uncongenial situation. In fact, he does this by becoming ill, or developing pain or other symptoms which make it impossible to carry on with what had become an intolerable situation. Thus, the child who is frightened of going to school, for perfectly reasonable reasons, if he does not just abscond, develops abdominal pain or may even come out in a rash. The adult for whom life is becoming too much may feel awful, get a headache or an asthmatic attack. The Victorians got the vapours when life became uncongenial; we now get 'stressed', but the mechanism is the same. This is not a conscious reaction; one does not say to oneself: 'Life is hell, I cannot stand my mother-in-law, I will get bilious and retreat respectably to bed.' One may or may not be aware of the fact that life or some aspect of it is ganging up, but the relationship between medical symptoms and the situation that has produced them is seldom realized.

The point to realize at the moment is that 'illness' is basically a reaction by the body to uncongenial circumstances. This reaction can take the form of a known disease like pneumonia or asthma or a headache, general malaise, irritability or agitation.

Symptoms are essentially a call for help and treatment; in our culture 'pain' and illness merit both sympathy and therapy. Equally they are an entirely acceptable reason to opt out of life. It is, on the whole, the patient who decides when he wants to stop — by retreating to bed or going to the surgery. Equally, it is basically he who decides when to go back although he may often take his doctor's (usually bad) advice and stay away longer than his natural inclinations or the strict needs of the situation. True malingering is rare, and this is itself a symptom of mental disturbance; all symptoms, be they psychic or somatic, are genuine and unconsciously motivated.

At this stage the reader may be tempted to say: 'This might explain some diseases, particularly stress and mental breakdown, but what about measles, typhoid, cancer and so on?' Space and the main subject of this book precludes a more detailed discussion of this fascinating topic except to say two things. Firstly, we do not yet know enough about the psychodynamics of the body's reaction to environmental challenge, to explain all illness in this way, and secondly, we do not have much idea as to what determines how the body will react. However, it is known that individuals tend to react differently to the same situational pressure. We can also cite plenty of examples of emotional states being expressed by physical bodily reactions — smiling, blushing, fear, alarm, and so on. The late menstrual period in the anxious girl, diarrhoea and a desire to pass water in the acutely anxious man, the rapidly beating heart in a crisis; these are all somatic reactions to emotional stress. We also know that all the body systems, chemical and hormonal, are controlled by the brain and that this includes immunity and resistance to disease.

The spectrum of disease is highly complex and a wide variety of factors, genetic, immunological, environmental, infective and so on, all enter into the picture. Obviously too, bacteria and viruses, chemicals and poisons all cause illness and exposure to these must play a part. But if 10 people are similarly exposed to influenza, infected meat pies, 30 cigarettes a day for 20 years, typhoid, cholera or polio, only a relatively small proportion of them will get 'infected'. What is it that determines survival or infection? Previous immunological protection from exposure plays some part, but this is far from the whole story. 'General resistance' and well-being are also factors. The individual's response to the environment is part of the picture which is, of course, psychosomatic.

The body mechanisms are controlled and coordinated by a variety of nervous and chemical systems. These originate in the brain and it is the total functioning of the brain which determines both personality and reaction. Disease could theoretically be mediated directly and indirectly through this system. Indeed, it must be.

Cancer represents a breakdown of cellular control in which a group of previously peaceful and well-behaved cells burst loose and become dangerous and parasitic mavericks. Cancer represents essentially a breakdown of the local control system. All sorts of things can contribute to individual cancers, including a genetic predisposition, but basically something has gone wrong with the internal control mechanisms to allow this to happen, which is a reflection of the well-being of the individual.

There are well-recorded 'miracle cancer cures' just as there are more frequent surgical, radiation and chemical cures. But the miracle or unexpected cure, be this from a visit to Lourdes, a faith healer, a change in diet or habitat, results in an alteration in the patient's attitude to his disease. This alters the body tone and may effect the cure. If the disease is not too advanced, survival may then ensue. In the same sort of way fatigue, anxiety, lack of exercise, the need for the tranquillizing effect of nicotine or alcohol can similarly play a part in determining resistance to other disease.

The importance attributed to trying to determine *why* a person is ill has already been emphasized. Particularly in the contexts just discussed, it is equally necessary to consider why certain people are never ill; what are the factors which delineate the healthy from the unhealthy?

Little is known about this at present, but if you, the reader, look around amongst your friends, colleagues and family, there is a fair chance that you will find that the happy, well-adjusted person who appears to have got his life 'about right', and has a wide range of interests, tends not to be ill. On the other hand, those who appear to 'enjoy ill health' may tend to have personality or behaviour disturbances, have chips rattling on their shoulders and be unfullfilled, perhaps over-ambitious and less than happy people.

All this is not to say that the treatment of illness is entirely psychotherapeutic, nor does it mean that all diseases will become treatable. Short-term conditions clearly respond well to drugs or surgery and if the stimulus is dealt with or, as so often is the case, is self-limiting, may not recur. Equally once physical change has occurred, as in arthritis, or a habit pattern established, as in asthma or migraine, it may be difficult to reverse. Drugs too can now affect the brain itself and depression, for instance, responds dramatically as may anxiety and tension.

Much more will be said about the problems of stress in Chapter 5. In medical terms, stress is the reaction which occurs in an individual when he can no longer meet the demands of the environment. Weak or inadequate people fold up easily and rapidly, any small upset or disappointment will phase them mentally or physically. Tough, robust people, whose morale tends to be high, seem indestructable but everyone has an ultimate breaking point, even if the way in which he breaks is unpredictable. One man's meat is another man's poison. I may be able to function well in one environment be this company, institution or family, and you, the reader, with more or less the same skills but a different personality, will fail to thrive. If, for instance, we swap bosses our reactions may well be reversed and the other one will become stressed.

What this philosophy adds up to is, first that mental health — and ill health, is as important as physical — indeed the two are inseparable. Second, that medicine, or in our immediate terms, executive health, involves what is coming to be called 'the whole man'. A full medical diagnosis depends on inquiry into, and assessment of, the individual in relation to his environment. This involves his work, his home and his leisure and social pursuits. The boss, the balance sheet and the union come home at the end of the day; just as the crying baby, the sleepless night, domestic stress and anxiety go to work in the morning.

This has been called the personality-environment equation: reasonable balance implies health, imbalance disease.

Of course, this really means that to understand and advise about executive health and executive diseases, one is essentially concerned about the way in which the executive lives and works. The climate within his organization, his home, his personality and his aspirations, what he does to relax: these are just as important as his aches and pains and his blood pressure. But in our view, his blood pressure and his cardiogram, his coronary proneness, are likely to be a reflection of his personality-environment equation.

The corollary of this approach is that we are inevitably interested in the company and the home, in the work group as well as the individual. This then is what this book will really be about. Managers create and manipulate environments, their health and that of their colleagues is likely to be a reflection of their success or failure. This will include fitting the right man into the right situation. It also involves a good match with wife or husband. The book will also include some basic medical information partly because it is hoped it should prove interesting and partly because it explains the remedial advice given. In any case, managers are used to taking decisions based on facts and figures. It may surprise them to know that in some branches of medicine we can now do the same — back the 'actuarial' odds to avoid a coronary. You will not win all the time but you might appreciably reduce the chances of losing.

PART ONE
MEDICAL HAZARDS

ONE

Life expectancy

Modern science and technology would have us believe that its marvels are making us live, if not for ever, at least for much longer. A glance at Figure 1:1 shows this not to be so. From 1840-1940 the life expectancy of a child of one (infant or neonatal mortality was very high in those days and many babies perished) went up from just below 50 to well over 60 and went on going up slowly until after the war. From 1950, however, it has hardly moved and the line on the graph has stayed nearly horizontal; the upper line represents women and the lower men.

Increased survival

Since the war, life expectancy has increased relatively little and at all ages women live longer than men. What has happened however, is that at all ages, more people are surviving. Hence, the population explosion. Figure 1:2 shows this growth and it is particularly worth noting the post-war increase in retired people. Projecting this forward to the end of the century shows that there will be well over ten million retired people in the population. This increase is facing western society with an entirely new problem, ie what to do with and how to integrate this important segment of the population who are currently more or less denied the right to work.

Leaving aside for the moment the toll that coronary heart disease takes of middle aged men, we can say that because of this trend the life expectancy of a man who achieves 65 in reasonable health is over 75, so that someone

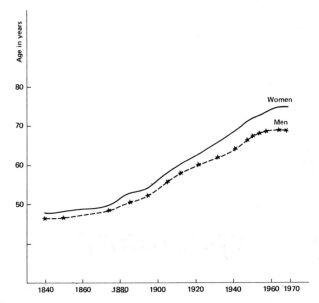

Figure 1:1 Expectation of life 1840-1970. (Source: Registrar General's figures for England and Wales)

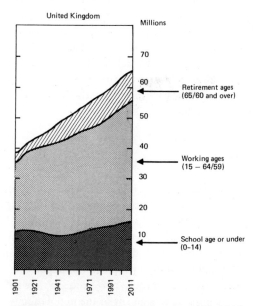

Figure 1:2 Population groups 1901-2011 showing relative proportions of school attenders, 'workers', retireds. (Source: Social Trends, No. 3, 1972, Central Statistical Office)

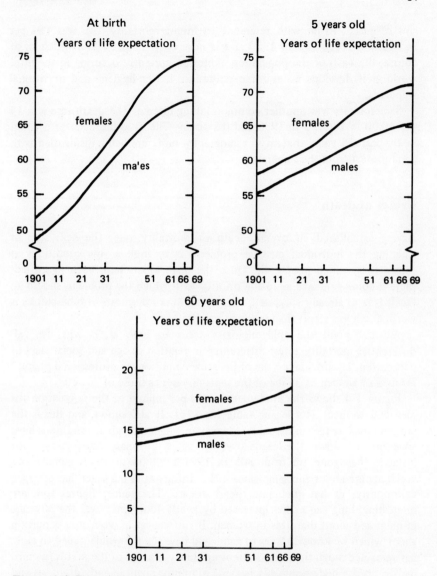

Figure 1:3 Expectation of life at birth, age 5 and age 60 in Great Britain. (Source: Social Trends, No. 3, 1973, Central Statistical Office)

retiring at 60 has to be able to support himself financially and emotionally for a good 15 years. Figure 1:3 shows the trends in life expectancy over this century.

As this type of epidemiological or statistical information is not widely understood, a few more figures about ourselves as a community, might not be out of place. Again with reference to infant mortality, this was 154 per *thousand* in 1850: 25 in 1950 and is now only 18 per 1000, which is, of course, the basis of the population explosion currently occuring in the third world as it develops water-borne sanitation, better hygiene and nutritional standards.

Tuberculosis was another common killing disease. The death rate was 14 per 10 00 in 1860: 3 in 1930 and 0.1 today. The drop has been so dramatic in the last 25 years that mass radiography units are being dismantled with great protest from their operators.

Causes of death

Having established an overall death or mortality rate, the next step in isolating the individual medical problems is to look at the conditions or causes from which people die. Once the main killers have been identified, there is some guidance as to the priority with which the problems should be tackled, ie as already suggested, the prevention or diagnosis of tuberculosis is worth much less effort than it was in say 1950.

Another point the epidemiologist needs to look at, is what we call differential mortality rates: differential in relation to age and social class or occupation. Do bricklayers die of the same conditions as professional people? Do men or women of 35 die of the same diseases as those of 70, etc.

Figure 1:4 shows the crude death rates per million of the population for men and women, as a league table for 1971. It also shows, and this is the most interesting fact in the table, the way in which individual conditions have gone up and down the league over the years. Coronary heart disease, for instance, has gone up from 805 in 1941 to 2603 in 1971; suicide and accidents are about the same since 1951. Influenza, a big killer, has dropped enormously, as has rheumatic heart disease. The cancer figures too, are interesting; lung cancer has increased by nearly four times over the 30 years in men, and more than this in women. Breast cancer in women, a condition about which we know little as to cause and have, on the whole, failed to cure, has remained much the same or crept up slowly. Cancer of the uterus (womb) has dropped a bit, presumably because of improvement in early diagnosis and more recently cervical cytology. Cancer is something which worries everyone; it is worth noting that in both sexes it is far from being the commonest cause of death, seldom being responsible for more than a third at any age or sex.

The next step in refining this understanding is to look at what is called age related mortality rates. The main details are shown in Figure 1:5 which shows three very significant points. The first is that at *all* ages women have a lower death rate than men. Why this should be, particularly through the child bearing age, has never been explained. Another interesting point here, is

Cause of death	Males				Females			
	1941	1951	1961	1971	1941	1951	1961	1971
Coronary heart disease	805	1 756	2 121	2 603	348	938	1 200	1 579
Cerebro vascular disease	1 228	1 378	1 394	1 309	1 262	1 734	1 925	1 948
Cancer of lung	230	550	871	1 060	48	91	139	224
Myocardial degeneration	2 144	1 710	860	891	1 982	2 129	1 301	879
Bronchitis	1 053	1 079	942	823	681	627	322	255
Pneumonia	849	578	634	733	553	496	637	885
Cancer of stomach	423	387	348	305	269	286	252	206
Road accidents	301	172	208	197	70	52	78	90
Rheumatic heart disease	259	194	154	108	307	298	233	172
Suicide	135	134	133	95	62	72	90	81
All causes	15 692	13 384	12 565	12 157	11 810	11 765	11 376	11 114

Figure 1:4 Crude death rates per million, all ages, and cause of death — top ten 1971. (Source: Registrar General's figures for England and Wales)

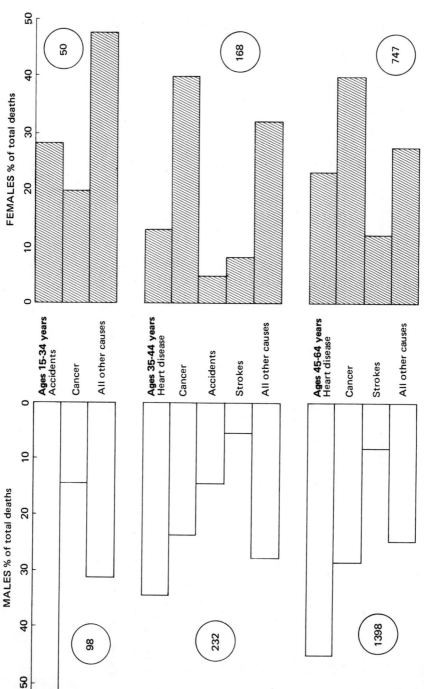

Figure 1:5 Principle causes of death for certain age groups in Great Britain. All the figures in circles represent total death rate per 100 000 (1970), all causes. (Source: based on Social Trends, No. 3, 1972, Central Statistical Office)

whether women who work — as might men — approximate more to men in their mortality figures. Accurate details are hard to get because work definitions on death certificates are not always accurate, especially for women, but there is a little evidence that they might. The probability is too that with an increase in smoking and other behavioural factors, death rates in women from coronary thrombosis and lung cancer are going up, but whether this is due to work, or boredom at home, is difficult to say.

The second point is that as one might expect, violence, accident and suicide are common causes of death in the young. The relative stability of middle age reduces the chances of violent death although, if one looked in more detail, suicide does creep back as a way out for older people.

The third and most important point is the overwhelming incidence of arteriosclerotic heart disease and 'other' cardiovascular disease. Coronary thrombosis and raised blood pressure are, together, far and away the biggest single cause of death in middle age. I say middle age advisedly because one is more concerned about surviving to 70 than about what one self or anyone else, dies of thereafter. Death is inevitable, the machinery wears out and what actually goes wrong — pump, body work or ignition — is of more marginal interest.

This may be summarized by saying that to survive into antiquity, firstly it is far better to be a woman, secondly, avoid violence and thirdly, try to avoid a coronary or raised blood pressure, which is the main theme of this book.

The last and unfortunately most difficult point to look at is mortality in relation to social class and occupation. Social classes I and II which include the professional and managerial groups, have nearly half the standardized mortality ratio of social class V, which is the poor and unskilled.

In fact, this is a very wide difference and shows a failure of our much vaunted health and welfare service to really deal with the problems. Over the last forty years, social classes I and II have always had an appreciably lower mortality ratio or greater life expectancy. The epidemiologists can break this type of information down into even finer detail and by plotting death rates and individual causes of death on a map, one could discover where not to live as well as what not to do. As might be expected, rural life is more conducive to survival than urban, and hard-water areas better than soft, from the point of view of avoiding coronary thrombosis.

Within this broad social class difference, it is interesting to look at individual diseases in men who do different jobs and for an obvious variety of reasons lead different lives. These are listed in Figure 1:6 which, although it looks intimidating, is of great social interest because basically it shows two things. First, that a lot of disease is sadly still related to standards of living, thus bronchitis is four times as common in class V as in class II, rheumatic fever four times and psychosis twice. The second, which is more encouraging, is that the diseases which are related to behaviour or early diagnosis like lung cancer (smoking), hypertension, cirrhosis (drinking) are lower in social classes I and II, ie they are beginning to learn about preventive medicine and how to live sensibly, to smoke less and control their weight, in a way that social classes IV and V have not yet achieved. Certainly doctors find that it is currently far more difficult to communicate with and persuade these groups to change their behavioural patterns. Chips with everything is an unbreakable habit.

Cause of death	Social classes		
	II	III	V
TB	54	96	185
Cancer	80	104	139
Lung cancer	72	107	148
Diabetes	103	100	122
Psychiatric	77	96	179
Rheumatic fever	67	85	207
IHD	95	106	112
Hypertension	96	99	138
Bronchitis	50	97	194
Cirrhosis	136	86	137
Suicide	94	87	184

Figure 1:6 Standardized mortality ratios for certain causes of death. The standard mortality ratio is a stastical index which gives deaths of a stated category — cause, age, sex, etc — as a percentage of expected deaths in the same period. Thus figures below 100 are better and those above 100 are worse than 'bogey' for the group. Social class II includes most managers, III includes skilled operators and V unskilled operators. (Source: Males 15-64, 1959-63, England and Wales, Registrar General's Decennial Supplement 1961)

Within each broad social class, it is difficult to get accurate figures about individual causes of death in relation to occupation. This is largely because of the difficulty of defining occupations on death certificates. The phrases company director, manager, business executive, etc, cover such a wide range of activities and tend to be misused. This can be seen from reading the law reports in almost any daily paper, where it can be observed that very dubious scrap merchants describe themselves as company directors. Also, many self-employed small shopkeepers are legitimately directors of their own limited company. Another difficulty is that the occupation on a death

Age	1959–63 Mean annual mortality per 100 000	1959–63 Per cent mortality compared to all men	1949–53 Per cent mortality compared to all men
25–34	61	54	102
35–44	145	60	80
45–54	468	66	92
55–64	1613	74	102
65–74 (including those who have retired)	4289	79	110

Figure 1:7 Executive mortality by age. (Source: BUPA Medical Centre)

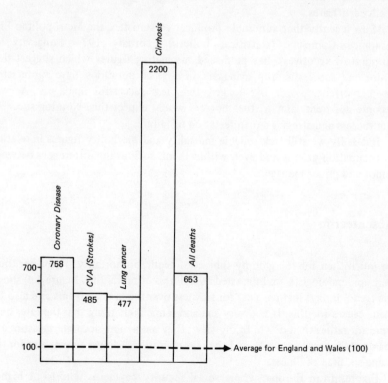

Figure 1:8 Company directors (1961 Census) aged 25-64. Ratio of actual deaths from selected causes to estimated number from taking all the England and Wales deaths (100 = standard)

certificate may be the one current at the time of death, ie a man may either be retired, or have drifted down into unskilled work in social class V, because he contracted lung disease as a miner.

Similarly it is difficult to get accurate information about the incidence of ischaemic heart disease (IHD) in managers, but there is some evidence that it is higher, particularly at a younger age, than in other working groups.

Sound statistics tend to be conflicting. Table 1.7 shows the relative incidence of IHD, stroke, lung cancer and cirrhosis between company directors and 'all men' in the population. IHD had seven, stroke five, lung cancer five and cirrhosis two thousand times the incidence. But it must be remembered that this refers to *relative* incidence within each disease group and that the overall incidence of cirrhosis, for instance, is very small. The last column in this table shows that the total death rate, up to age 65, was 6½ times that of the average. But these figures must be qualified, firstly, by the fact that they go back to 1961, and secondly, that as ahs already been said, the so called directors were probably a polyglot group, defined purely from death certificates.

More recently that admirable producer of statistics, the Metropolitan Life Insurance Company (statistical bulletin February 1974 Longevity of Corporate Executives), has published fascinating figures which suggest that senior and successful 'top managers' in large corporations, have appreciably lower mortality — or live longer, than less successful managers. As will become apparent later in thes book, I would expect this. Nothing succeeds like success and stress is a manifestation of failure.

But sadly we still lack reliable mortality and morbidity figures in relation to occupation groups and even within them, such as the differences between senior and junior managers.

Absenteeism

So much then for the gloomy subject of death, or mortality. The other thing that epidemiologists are interested in is illness or morbidity. Figure 1:9 shows the trend of days lost per year for sickness over the last few years and also the main causes for this. It is a very sad and remarkable thing that the rates have gone up rather than down. In my view, they are a more accurate measure of a man's willingness to work, and the community's readiness to pay him for not doing so, than of illness.

Figures from Europe, where social security payments tend to be higher, are even more frightening. The late Harold Winncott wrote one of his most perceptive articles on this subject in *The Financial Times*. It was called 'A week off to tile the bathroom' and related how a Coventry car worker got a week off with backache and earnings related benefit to tile his bathroom, in which activity he made a good net gain.

Executive work is physically undemanding and partly because of this managers, in my view, tend to take too little rather than too much time off work. So indispensable do they feel, that they must drag themselves in to

	1955/56	1967/68
Respiratory disease	27.21	36.41
Accidents, violence, poisonings	10.79	19.66
Digestive disorders	16.29	19.04
Arthritis and joint trouble	12.06	16.92
Heart disease	11.54	16.59
Mental disorders	5.32	8.29
Totals	83.21	116.91

Figure 1:9 Millions of days off work due to specific illnesses (short-term incapacity). (Source: Whitehead, T P., *Journal of the Royal Society of Medicine* **65, 567, 1972)**

	25–34	35–44	45–54	55–64	All ages
All males (excluding spells of 3 days or less)	5.8	7.1	9.8	18.4	8.9
Directors (all included)	1.7	3.9	3.7	6.3	4.7

Figure 1:10 Means days off work / year. (Sources: Ministry of Pensions and National Insurance 'Report on an inquiry into the incidence of incapacity for work', 1961-62, HMSO 1965; IOD Questionnaire)

make sure that everyone else in the office shares their colds and 'flu. Comparative figures are given in Figure 1:10.

In general medical terms, these figures show that quite different conditions cause lost time from those that cause death. Mental illness causes about 10 per cent of absenteeism and an insignificant number of deaths. This then is how the epidemiologist tells us what conditions or areas we ought to worry about and sets our priorities for dealing with the problems in the right order.

In national terms, there is an urgent need to do something about the welfare state disease of 'unwillingness to work' reflected in strikes and so called sickness. This is a political rather than a medical problem, because the doctors quite rightly protest that it is not their job to tell a patient that he does not have backache and consequently could go back to work.

Every company should carry out its own departmental epidemiology. If this is done, by say the personnel department, two things will probably become apparent. Firstly, that a high proportion of the absenteeism is experienced by a small proportion of the staff. Within this, it may well be found that a previously good attender has run into a bad patch. Probably something has gone wrong with his/her life pattern and he/she can no longer cope. By identifying those concerned, steps can be taken to deal with them.

Secondly, the rate will be found to vary from department to department and this is usually a function of low morale, bad interpersonal relations or supervision.

But as far as the business group is concerned, there is no shadow of doubt that cardiovascular disease — coronary thrombosis and raised blood pressure — is the biggest single problem, which is why most of this book is devoted to telling readers how to try and avoid it.

TWO

Coronary Thrombosis

We saw in the last chapter that coronary thrombosis (to be referred to as IHD, ischaemic heart disease) was the main killer of middle-aged men before retirement. I joined the Institute of Directors in 1958 with a brief to see if there were any occupational health problems related to the member's way of life and, if so, whether he could be helped to deal with them.

In those days rather little was known about the factors which predisposed to coronary artery disease, although it was believed to be a social class I and II disease, related primarily to a sedentary life. I became something of a medical heretic, because I preached the prevention of this condition at a time when doctors as a whole thought this a waste of time.

The information we collected soon confirmed the fact that not only was IHD the number one killer, but also that many of the predisposing factors seemed specifically related to the businessman's way of life. We were also amused to find that there were no figures whatever to support the then popular contention that duodenal ulcer was the disease *par excellence* of the harassed executive. One seldom saw 'ulcerated men' as patients and the statistics seldom referred to them. The probability was that because their American counterparts got ulcers, perhaps from too many dry Martinis, the successful British copy had to have the same illnesses.

Figure 2:1 shows the way in which overall death rates from IHD have been going up since the end of the war for those under retiring age. The upper line refers to men aged 35-64 and the lower to those between 45 and 54 — more or less the prime of life.

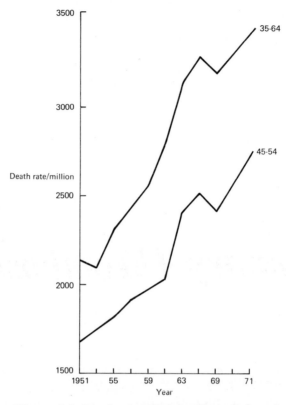

Figure 2:1 Death rates in men from ischaemic heart disease

| Year | Sex | AGE | | | | All ages |
		25–	45–	65–	75+	
1940	M	80	1 446	4 432	6 570	808
1957	M	221	3 240	11 555	18 972	2 208
1962	M	307	4 051	13 946	25 145	2 767
1965	M	367	4 525	14 661	27 284	2 982
1971	M	359	4 823	16 278	35 276	3 501
1940	F	20	425	2 165	3 759	374
1957	F	28	805	5 201	10 989	1 226
1962	F	42	1 007	6 126	15 341	1 657
1965	F	55	1 090	6 437	16 246	1 801
1971	F	51	1 172	6 793	23 613	2 394

Figure 2:2 Death rates per million living from arteriosclerotic heart disease, including coronary risk, by age and sex. (Source: Registrar General's figures for England and Wales)

Figure 2:2 gives the age-related totals for IHD and hypertension and from this one can make the generalization that nearly a third of all businessmen will die before reaching the age of 65. The community, their companies and their families will lose them. It is because I believe so firmly that, given early detection of vulnerable people, much of this waste of life can be prevented, we have built up The Medical Centre and continue to hammer away at risk factors. Successful prevention, of course, implies that the vulnerable person, having been identified, is then willing to mend his ways and alter his way of life.

What is coronary thrombosis?

The heart is a muscular pump whose job it is to continuously pump blood around the body. It is very similar to the circulation pump in a central heating system, which also has to adjust itself to fluctuations in demand and variations in temperature.

Basically, the heart muscle behaves in the same way and has the same requirements as all the other muscles in the body. Thus it works better if it is kept in training and does not like being flabby and infiltrated with fat. Similarly too, the muscle, although filled with blood on the inside, has to have its own blood supply and this it gets through the *coronary arteries,* so called because they run round the heart rather like a crown. The two, right and left coronary arteries, arise from the aorta (which is the main artery or 'blood supply main') taking blood from the heart to the rest of the body, just beyond the valves which control the outward flow of blood.

The coronaries are perfectly normal arteries and are prone to all diseases of the arterial or cardiovascular system. One of these is called arteriosclerosis or hardening of the arteries. With increasing age, partly as a result of normal wear and tear and possibly as a reaction to raised blood pressure (discussed later), the walls of the artery thicken and lose their flexibility. In the larger arteries, the walls may actually calcify and be visible on x-ray. This gross form of hardening used to be known as pipe-stem arteries, because they looked (remotely) like a clay pipe stem.

As well as walls which harden and thicken, arteries, and veins (less important here), have a thin smooth shining endothelial lining which functions firstly, to promote the easy and smooth flow of blood and secondly, to allow 'wanted substances' to diffuse through the lining. If this endothelium becomes damaged, it gets roughened and sets up local turbulence, which may collect blood clot; this in turn increases the roughening and reduces the calibre of the vessel. It is known now that one of the causes of this reduction in calibre or damage to the lining of the artery is the deposition of a fatty substance called cholesterol, in the layers under the lining. This is why the excess of fat in the blood and diet is so important in the genesis of IHD.

As a vessel, particularly if it is relatively small, becomes narrowed, the flow of blood becomes reduced and slowed down. The mechanism that controls blood clotting is immensely complicated, but obviously if the blood did not clot when it escaped from the vacsular system, bleeding to death would result, as happens in fact, in haemophilia, the bleeding disease. In practice, it is the stimulus of tissue damage — usually by injury — that stimulates blood clotting and scab formation. To a degree, this is what happens within the arteries when blood flow is slowed or stopped. Similarly blood in a test tube will clot without an anticoagulant.

Thus it is easy to understand why damage or disease of the artery wall, and reduction in circulation rate, causes the blood within the artery to clot. This, of course, blocks the vessel and this blockage is known medically as a *thrombosis.* Coronary thrombosis is, therefore, blockage of the arteries to the heart by blood clot.

If blood cannot get through an artery, the region or part supplied by it is denied its nutritional supply and dies or is damaged. Consequently, blocking of the blood supply to part of the heart or the brain may cause serious tissue damage or death. Coronary or cerebral thrombosis results from disease of the artery wall (arteriosclerosis) and to a lesser extent from upset of the clotting system.

The coronary arteries have two peculiarities not shared with other arteries. The first is that they are end arteries. This means that unlike the digestive system, for instance, there is very little overlap between the areas supplied by each artery. Thus, if an artery or its branch is blocked, the muscle supplied will die because it has no alternative source of blood. This makes the heart almost uniquely vulnerable to thrombosis. The muscle supplied by a blocked coronary artery dies and the heart may cease to function. The other difference is that although arteriosclerosis is a generalized disease coming on largely with age, the coronary arteries become diseased much earlier and often well before the larger arteries are involved. Thus in younger people, say under 55, IHD can be an isolated disease whereas in the older group, it is very much part of a general wear and tear process.

Recent post-mortem studies, firstly on American soldiers killed in Korea and later on very young children, have shown that atheroma (the name given to cholesterol deposits) are found very early in life in the coronary arteries. Thus it could be that childhood diet including too much animal fat plays a significant part in determining the disease.

To summarize: coronary thrombosis is due to the blockage of diseased coronary arteries by blood clot. The muscle area deprived of its blood supply dies, and if this is extensive enough so does the person, as the heart can no longer function.

Death results from two main causes: not enough muscle left to keep the heart pumping and sudden disorganization of the heart's rythmic control mechanism by the damage. This is the type of condition which can be so dramatically dealt with by the electric gadgetry of a modern intensive care unit. By using electrodes and pacemakers, the heart can be kept going literally until it has sorted itself out. Similarly, in more chronic conditions in which the control mechanism is out of order, long-term pacemakers can be successfully used to keep up a normal rhythm.

After a coronary thrombosis, the muscle is replaced by scar tissue and becomes quite firm. If there is a large scarred area which flaps about rather weakly, it can sometimes be plicated surgically, to the benefit of cardiac function.

It has now been realized that in rehabilitating a 'coronary heart' it is better to be active rather than passive. It is both safe and desirable to build up the remaining muscle to increase both its strength and its blood supply.

The coronary arteries also suffer from arteriosclerosis without thrombosis, particularly in a heart enlarged by hypertension (discussed later). In this case, there is enough blood to supply the muscle at rest, but not the greater demands of activity. When a muscle cannot get enough blood on which to work, it rebels and causes pain which, of course, stops the demand. Heart pain on exercise of this type is called angina of effort and is a relatively common condition. A man walking to work will always have to stop at the same place and rest until the pain has worn off. Such pain, which may go down the left arm, is relieved by TNT tablets which have the capacity to dilate the blood vessels and increase the blood supply. Cramp in athletes and claudication in the legs is due to similar causes.

Some angina is stable and people can live for years with it, other types are more progressive and lead to heart failure or fatal thrombosis.

Surgical efforts are currently being devoted to plastic operations to replace damaged vessels or 'ream' out the existing ones. So far they are not more than experimental, but some of the results are promising.

The heart and blood pressure

An interesting example of the gaps in our knowledge about important medical things is that we still do not fully understand what causes certain types of hypertension — high blood pressure. There is a chicken and egg situation in that it is a simple law of hydraulics that if the calibre of a pipe is reduced, the pressure to maintain the same circulation must be raised, and we do not yet know which happens first in hypertension.

It is also known medically that if blood pressure goes up significantly the arteries react to this by becoming hard, rigid and narrower. There are thus two possible explanations of hypertension. Firstly, that the heart goes mildly berserk and works at a raised pressure, to which the arteries respond by becoming 'sclerotic' or secondly, that narrowing of the arteries demands a greater output from the heart.

Two other factors come into this picture. One is that certain organs like the kidney have a priority demand for blood supply to maintain their essential service of getting rid of waste products, which would otherwise build up and poison the system. If the kidney becomes diseased, as in nephritis, its vessels get narrowed and the need to maintain an adequate kidney blood supply puts up the general blood pressure, which is why chronic kidney disease is a common cause of hypertension and one that is always looked for. The second factor is that as arteriosclerosis is a normal wear and tear age change, blood pressure tends to go up with age in order to keep up an adequate circulation through furred up pipes.

The detailed mechanisms that control blood pressure and distribution and the way in which supply and demand are equated, eg what happens when one starts running for a bus, are complicated and need not be described here. Mostly they are mediated through the autonomic nervous system, and some modern drugs which are effective in controlling blood pressure act by influencing or altering this part of the control system.

Clearly, raised blood pressure will affect both the heart and the blood vessels. As to the heart, it has to work harder to keep up the circulation. Its muscle hypertrophies, as it does to a lesser extent in the trained athlete, and the heart enlarges. Sooner or later, however, the overworked heart gives up and goes into failure. The coronary arteries, of course, share in the generalized arteriosclerosis which adds to the risk of failure.

Other more local conditions like a leaking valve (as in rheumatic heart disease), a narrowed main artery or holes in the heart, all of which reduce the output of the heart, lead to hypertrophy, hypertension and heart failure. Many of these conditions, particularly the holes in the heart which will lead to a mixture of arterial and venous blood in 'blue babies', can be dealt with successfully by modern surgery. Holes are repaired, valves replaced and arteries mended, with, on the whole, admirable results.

When the heart fails, blood builds up on the input or venous side and there is a tendency to waterlogging and breathlessness because of inadequate oxygenation. Similarly, disease or upset in the lungs, which have a low pressure circulation system designed to oxygenate venous blood, will upset the heart, and failure to oxygenate puts up the blood pressure and pulse rate.

As to the blood vessels, they develop arteriosclerosis which leads to a tendency either to block or burst. Reduction of blood supply to the legs, for instance, means that the powerful leg muscles become starved and cannot work. They react in the same way as the heart and cause cramp-like pain called intermittent claudication; intermittent because it is work related. Total blockage obviously leads to death of the tissue supplied, usually toes or the lower leg. This is called gangrene and mostly necessitates amputation. Blockage of vessels in the brain, caused by thrombosis, constitutes one form of stroke and clearly interferes with cerebral function often shown as paralysis of one or other side of the body. Another form of stroke is when a weakened vessel bursts through being unable to stand up to the raised pressure. This produces a cerebral haemorrhage with damage to the brain by the leakage of blood. Vessels elsewhere can bulge (aneurism) and leak, as a result of prolonged hypertension.

Life is dependent on the complicated interrelationship between brain, heart and lungs and it is said that there are really only two ways of dying – from either heart or respiratory failure. But a lot of things can cause either of these. All three systems have tremendous reserve capacity which can be developed by training and regular use, and protected by reducing demand, as in not being overweight. Lastly, of course, there is a very close relationship between emotional states and the heart. Fear, anxiety, tension, etc, all influence the heart. Just as behavioural situations like smoking and fatigue influence function, so does personality and emotion. To a degree, coronary thrombosis and hypertension must be personality-related or psychosomatic diseases.

Coronary risk factors

Most diseases are caused by the presence (eg virus, bacteria, toxin) or absence (eg vitamin, protein, mineral) of single identifiable factors. Unfortunately, IHD is what we call multifactorial in its causation. This means that not one, but a number of possible factors contribute to its causation. This situation is made more complicated by the problem that the way in which the factors operate varies from person to person, or even possibly from time to time in the same person.

Thus, some heavy cigarette smokers survive without getting either IHD or lung cancer and others succumb relatively early or quickly. This variation in the way in which the 'multifactors' operate is a nuisance in another important scientific way. It makes the statistical assessment of the effects of altering one of the factors extremely difficult, which is why it is so hard to 'prove' that people live longer by cutting smoking or taking more exercise. By altering one of these, the life style changes considerably and the effect on the heart is, for better or worse, more complicated than the mere withdrawal of nicotine or an increase in muscle and blood supply.

However, over the last ten years or so, a number of elegant epidemiological exercises have convincingly isolated individual factors which undoubtedly contribute to coronary proneness. These are called coronary risk factors.

Various trials are now in hand to demonstrate an increase in life expectancy or reduction in morbidity by reforming the way of life of groups of people and comparing what happens to them with an unreformed or control group.

The earliest of these attempts was the New York Anti-Coronary Club, which I visited in 1968. Over several years, they persuaded men to live on what they euphemistically called a prudent (and very boring) diet, but they did show that the 'treated group' did better than the imprudent or untreated group. Subsequently, other trials and figures have confirmed this.

Working along these lines, it is now possible to list a number of known risk factors. If an individual is then measured for the presence or absence of such factors one can strike a balance and rate his risk as would an insurance underwriter, which, in a modified way, is what insurance companies do.

In various and variable ways, from person to person, the following factors are currently believed to influence an individual's chances of getting IHD.

Genetic

In ordinary social terms, we hear about long-lived families and, clearly if this is true, the propensity towards longevity must be genetically determined and 'inherited'. This does not mean that every member of the family will automatically live to a ripe old age but it does mean that, other things being equal, they are more likely to.

The converse is equally true: there are also short-lived families, but one hears less about these. Their members tend to die young, because of inherited diseases or predispositions, which 'kill them off early'. IHD is one of them and we now know that both fathers and surprisingly, more particularly mothers, pass a propensity for IHD on to their children. Figure 2:3 shows the increased mortality rate from IHD in first degree relatives for male and female coronary patients. And they are quite alarming.

Unfortunately, this inheritance is not transmitted in a simple way, like for instance the gene for haemophilia (the bleeding disease). In practice, there are a number of 'family ways' in which IHD and high blood pressure is caused. One of the most interesting of these is called familial hypercholesterolaemia. In this, for genetically determined metabolic reasons, blood lipids (fat) are very high and lead to early death from atherosclerosis. This is so serious that babies born to mothers known to have the condition are now tested at birth and put on to special 'artery protecting diets'.

Inheritance also acts in a secondary way through what are called shared environmental factors. Some years ago, the Americans showed that wives (who in any case have a much lower IHD rate than their husbands) who were married to coronary husbands, had themselves an increased IHD rate, ie there was something in their joint way of life which increased the risk.

Children inevitably share the physical and mental environment of their parents and, to a degree, this must affect their life expectancy. Here are two simple examples. The first refers to smoking and drinking. For obvious reasons, it is far more difficult to stop the children of parents who smoke cigarettes from themselves smoking. 'Mum and Dad do, why shouldn't I?' Similarly, the amount of alcohol consumed is part of a family pattern and in

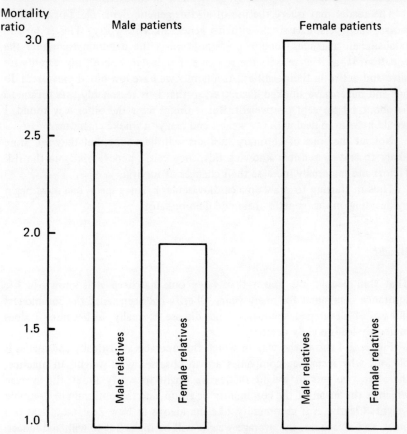

Figure 2:3 **Family history and ischaemic heart disease. Relatives of 200 patients with ischaemic heart disease. (Source: Dr Joan Slack)**

France and Italy, where alcohol is cheap and traditionally consumed, drinking is also a national cultural and very dangerous pattern. More people die of cirrhosis although there are fewer drunks to be seen in the street than in England.

The second concerns obesity. It is now believed that fat babies make fat children who make fat adults. Interesting too, at all ages fat individuals are far less physically active than their lean counterparts. Although body build (the tall, thin, active and manic ectomorph, the muscular mesomorph, the pear drop, obese endomorph) is genetically determined, eating habits are determined by the family pattern.

In America, where the consumption of carbohydrate-rich convenience foods, soft drinks and ice cream is unreasonably high, if not alarming, the incidence of obesity is frightening, particularly in children.

The reader may query the use of all this genetic rigmarole. For better or worse, each person is stuck with his genes, so why worry? This is far too fatalistic an attitude. Genetic predisposition is the denominator under the equation. It, as it were, sets the risk rate. For instance, both my parents are alive and active in their eighties. As a family we have low blood pressure. I do not and never have smoked cigarettes, so that it is reasonably safe for me to be about 10 per cent overweight. But if things were the other way round, I would be wise to deal with my weight and crazy to smoke cigarettes.

Not all the sons of coronary mothers will die young, but they are more likely to and by sensibly knowing this, they can, I believe, mitigate the risk factors and materially increase their chances of survival.

Thus in starting to draw up a cardiovascular balance sheet, one must begin by deciding on the 'genetic or family' denominator.

Weight

That thin people live longer than fat people has been well known to life insurance companies for many years. Obesity has been called the commonest disease of developed countries, and disease it really is because it does indirectly lead to early death.

Figure 2:4 shows the way in which this operates statistically and makes it obvious why insurance companies are so obsessed with weight. In practice, there are two sets of weight figures we ought to worry about, the average which is the mean of the community or group, and the optimum or desirable weight. Clearly, if a community like the Maoris in New Zealand all eat too much and are obese, the average weight will be high. But so will, and indeed is, their mortality rate. Thus, as averages go up like the cost of living, for survival, we need to keep our eye on a lower optimum weight which has to be calculated by using life tables based on survivors rather than averages.

Obesity is, in fact, a classical example of how interrelated multifactorial factors, in practice are. Fat people are physically inactive; there is just too much of them to rush about. They tend to tolerate or even to stoke up their obesity for basic personality reasons. A lot of seriously fat people, for instance, are sadly insecure and overeat for comfort. But, in addition to this, fat people have much higher blood pressures than thin people and obviously are more likely to have raised blood fat. Thus, there are several good reasons why a fat person (and ten or more per cent over 'bogey' is the start point for obesity) is likely to be coronary prone.

Figure 2:4 shows the way in which life insurance companies work out the loading for overweight people. Mortality rate goes up 13 per cent for 10 per cent overweight, 25 per cent for 20 per cent and a vast 42 per cent for 30 or more per cent overweight. Stated starkly like this, it can easily be understood

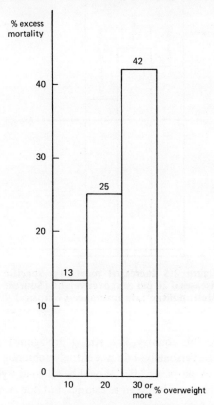

Figure 2:4 Increased mortality due to obesity (excess). (Source: Metropolitan Life Insurance Company)

why obesity is such a serious disease, and, of course, one that is delightfully or miserably easy to cure – by eating less.

Figure 2:5 shows the medical reasons why obese people die sooner, the incidence of heart disease, cerebral stroke or diabetes is all appreciably greater. It is also said that accidents and suicide are commoner in fat people because they tend to be unhappy.

There are those who believe that individual dietary factors like animal fat and sugar intake also, and independently, determine coronary proneness.

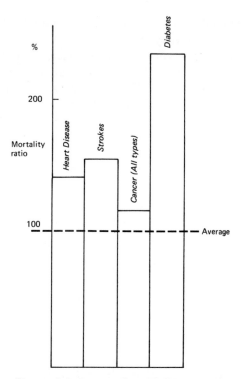

Figure 2:5 Increased mortality: specific diseases if 20 per cent overweight. (Source: Metropolitan Life Insurance Company)

Professor Yudkin, in this country, is a strong protagonist of refined sugar being a 'cause' of IHD. Personally, I do not entirely subscribe to this view and think that for ordinary purposes, 'diet' should be taken as a general reflection of weight. Thus, alcohol can be taken as calories, but not as well as bread and potatoes.

Blood Lipids (fat) — Cholesterol and Triglycerides

Figure 2:6 shows the now well-established relationship between raised blood cholesterol and IHD. All other things being equal, which, of course, they never entirely are, the man with a significantly raised cholesterol has at least twice the chance of getting a coronary than someone with lower levels.

Since the cholesterol story was established, much more has been learnt about other fats in the blood which are related to cholesterol. In fact, it is usually raised triglycerides which cause the trouble. But here this distinction need not concern the general reader.

Although overweight people tend to have higher cholesterol and triglyceride levels than do thin people, this is far from always being the case. Many normal weighted people have levels raised enough to need attention. But, obviously, in dealing with a cholesterol problem, the first and simplest thing is to deal with weight.

At the beginning of the chapter we noted that 'cholesterol' contributes to atherosclerosis by becoming deposited under the lining of the blood vessels.

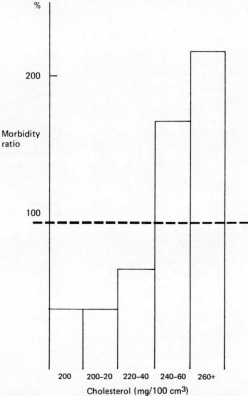

Figure 2:6 Cholesterol and heart disease. (Source: Framingham Community Study USA)

The milky white patches which this causes in the larger vessels were called atheroma, giving the name to the condition. Chemically, cholesterol is related to the steroid hormones and through this is related to the multifactorial causation of IHD. We now know that people constantly under pressure, who are stressed, tend to have raised cholesterol. During a period of considerable personal stress, which led to missing a holiday one year, my cholesterol went up to nearly 300. When I came back from a month's holiday and remarriage, it came down to 240.

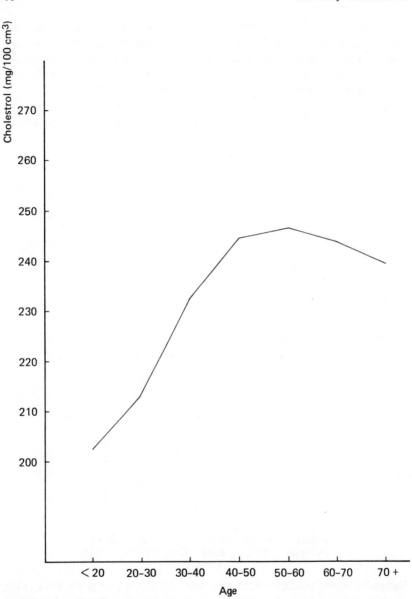

Figure 2:7 Mean cholesterol by age in men. (Source: BUPA Medical Centre)

Many years ago I looked after the six senior directors who had built up a then medium sized engineering company. Although not young, they were in reasonable order when first seen. Two years later they all looked very worn and tired, and four out of the six had appreciably raised cholesterols. When all this was put to the chairman, he made the point that not only had the company gone briefly into the red but that it was also expanding considerably. Knowing the chairman and directors very well by this time, I made my point which was that this group was under too much pressure and perhaps they needed underpinning, so that they could direct rather than manage. This was done and all went back to normal. I believe that they have all now retired.

Figure 2:7 shows mean cholesterol values in relation to age. It will be seen that the line reaches a peak between the ages of 50 and 60 and then appears to fall. This fall is illusory because what in fact happens is that the men with high cholesterol levels die off, leaving the 'low-level' survivors with a much reduced mean value, as shown on the graph. What occurs is that sadly IHD sorts the cohort into two separate groups or populations: the living and the dead. Hence the need to identify and treat vulnerable people.

Males		IHD	Cancer	All causes
Period 1	Hospital N (diet)	5.72	2.76	34.56
	Hospital K (control)	15.18	3.43	40.20
Period 2	Hospital K (diet)	7.50	7.28	35.12
	Hospital N (control)	12.97	4.50	38.78
		$p < 0.002$	NS	NS

Figure 2:8 Age adjusted death rates (causes per 1000 person years). (Source: Miettinen, M. Turpeinen, O. *et al,. Lancet,* ii, 7782, 1972)

Figure 2:8 shows some interesting figures from Finland, where over many years, the patients in two long-stay hospital populations were used to study the effect of diet on IHD and other diseases. In period 1 hospital N had a low cholesterol diet and hospital K the normal one. IHD rate was 5.72 in N and three times this in K. Switching the diets reversed the effect, thus demonstrating a marked relationship between diet and IHD rate. By implication too, it demonstrates the value of modifying diet.

The blood lipids are both fussed about and measured because they do seem to be one of the most critical factors in IHD, but also because it is now possible to deal successfully with cholesterol by diet or by drugs. Anybody with significantly raised lipids, who does not treat them seriously, should be regarded as a suicide!

We know, for instance, that given proper treatment, some of the deposit gets 'washed' out of the artery walls. And by feeding polyunsaturated (vegetable) fats as distinct from saturated (animal) fats, consistently, the balance of body fat can be altered away from the dangerous end of the spectrum.

People with raised cholesterol should minimize their consumption of animal fat and dairy products such as cream, milk and butter. Margarines such as Flora or Outline, skimmed milk, and vegetable oil for cooking are the alternatives, and they soon become bearable.

Exercise

It is now well established that sedentary people have a higher IHD rate than physically active people. The classical demonstration of this was the difference in the rates between drivers and conductors in London Transport buses. Other similar figures have been obtained from other work groups and are shown in Figure 2:9.

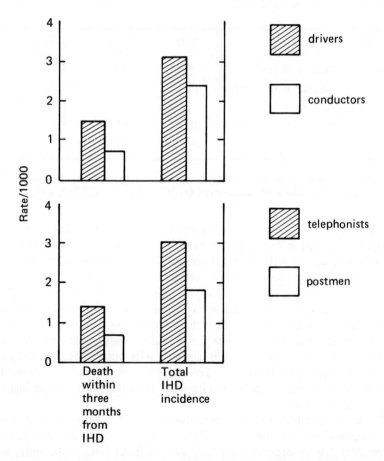

Figure 2:9 Examples of the difference in IHD rates between sedentary and physically active people. (Source: Morris, J.N. *et al.)*

The reasons why the physically fit heart is a better proposition than the fat-infiltrated flabby heart were given in the introductory section of this chapter. It has been established that while fit people may not always have a lower coronary rate, they certainly stand up to the result of the thrombosis better. Their hearts have a better cardiac reserve.

But the heart apart, the exercise that goes towards the establishment of reasonable fitness has other values as well. Taking regular exercise after middle age is a discipline which has its own virtues. Spending 30 or so minutes a day in this way means that this is time not spent at work or worrying. Fit people are more alert and active and there is some evidence to suggest that they are intellectually more effective and may sleep better. I suspect too that fit people stand up to fatigue and periods of stress rather better than do the flabby.

Muscles are made to be used and, if kept in 'well-oiled' use, will go on remaining strong and useful until late in life. Similarly, joints remain mobile if they are regularly exercised. Physical fitness is a life preserver in more ways than one, interestingly, patients who have had a coronary thrombosis are now got rapidly out of bed and very soon put on to a regime of graded exercise. The undamaged heart muscle must be kept fit, and then developed to replace what has been lost.

Incidentally, it is fairly easy to build exercise into one's life, starting as an attitude of mind. Walk some of the way to work, walk upstairs and do not get 'stuck in the lift', go and see people rather than make them come to you. All this can add up to a lot of exercise. But do not be misguided into thinking that exercise loses weight. It does burn up a few calories, but not that many. The post-rugby beer puts most of it back and it used to be said that one had to walk from London to Brighton to work off a large city dinner.

Cigarettes

Choose your poison proclaim the anti-smoking advertisements as I write this. Cigarette smoking is still on the increase and it is lethal as shown by the statistics in Figure 2:10. This figure illustrates the difference in death rates (per 100 000) between male smokers aged 45-64 and 65-79 and non-smokers. It is striking that for all the common causes listed, smokers have at least twice the death rate of non-smokers. For lung cancer, it is far more than this. In addition, there is the morbidity rate, not shown here, of chronic bronchitis. How, after seeing figures like this, any sane person can go on smoking cigarettes, is a mystery to me.

Nicotine is a very remarkable drug. Much of the basic physiological research on the working of the autonomic nervous system was done with nicotine which paralyses one set of the nerve ganglia.

Nicotine is both effective as a tranquillizer and also highly addictive, probably more so than 'pot' or alcohol, and, almost certainly, it does more serious damage than both. But sadly perhaps it does not cause enough socially aberrant behaviour, as the others do, to make the community take action. In addition, the revenue income from tobacco makes it virtually impossible for any government to seriously discourage smoking.

Some years ago, it was my misfortune to try to advise a very self-centred, indulgent young man. One year he had taken to smoking again and there were serious changes in his cardiograph. I showed him the two sets of tracings and said that the deterioration was due to 'filter tips'. He stopped and remains alive. His cardiograph returned to normal.

Smoking a cigarette, apart from calming the nerves, puts up the pulse rate and blood pressure, which is not good for hypertensive people, also it

Cause of death	Age 45-64		Age 65-79	
	Smokers	Never	Smokers	Never
All causes	1329	708	5196	3642
All cancer	267	125	973	555
Lung cancer	87	11	262	23
All heart and circulatory	802	422	3238	2471
IHD	615	304	2159	1586

Figure 2:10 Death rates (per 100 000) of smokers versus non-smokers. (Source: National (United States) Cancer Institute Monograph, No. 19, Hammond Study)

liberates adrenalin, which in turn liberates glucose. This is why stopping smoking often produces a craving for sugar: it raises the carbon monoxide level in the blood which damages the lining of the vessels and may start off atheroma. It is probable that the 20-30 a day man has a steady 10-15 per cent carbon monoxide level; by the evening his head is metaphorically pretty close to an old-fashioned gas oven.

The increased IHD risk in smokers is by far the most cogent reason for not smoking cigarettes. And for some of the reasons already listed, improvement starts the moment you stop; 30 000 men under 65 die every year from IHD as against *1000* in an older age group from lung cancer.

The statistics in Figure 2:11 show smoking rates for various occupational groups. It will be seen that men coming to The Medical Centre have a smoking incidence of about 40 per cent. Sadly, it seems that although probably fewer people are smoking, those that do so, smoke more. This is particularly true of the young.

We manage to persuade 24 per cent of the people who come to us to give up or reduce smoking, largely by showing them these figures. Thus, if you are a smoker, the 'non-smokers' club, is one you should join at once. The statistics are shown in Figure 2:12.

Inhaling the tar-containing cigarette smoke is micro or personal air pollution in a big way. The lungs are, if you like, constantly in a smoke-filled room and they want to cough and splutter. Because inhaled smoke is irritant and also, of course, because more is absorbed from the lungs than the mouth, there is a likelihood that the lung tissue will become irritated, inflamed and later destroyed by the constant, irritant assault of inhalation. This is, in fact,

Social class	1958 %	1965 %	1971 %
II	58	54	43
III	60	53	53
V	61	59	59

Figure 2:11 Cigarette smokers by social class.
(Source: Tobacco Research Council)

Given up	Reduced 30% or more	Started or increased 30% or more	No change	Total number
13%	11%	7%	69%	1493

Figure 2:12 Percentage change in cigarette smoking habit at first follow-up visit (in smokers only). (Source: BUPA Medical Centre)

what happens. Smokers cough leads to chronic bronchitis known abroad as the English disease, to which our climate contributes, leading to breathlessness, and heart and respiratory failure. Chronic bronchitis is the biggest single cause of lost time in this country and most of it is due to smoking.

In my view, and I am not a cancer expert, lung cancer is more a reflection of the irritation-infection cycle that follows smoking, than it is of direct carcinogenic stimulation caused by the tars. If the tars really were all that carcinogenic, a much higher lung cancer rate in smokers would be expected, such as occurs with other carcinogens. The surprising thing, too, is that some smokers get by without coughing and others do not.

So there is a wide personal sensitivity. Coronaries apart, coughers should certainly stop while they have still some lung left. We know too that in other parts of the body where chronic irritation leads to the constant removal and replacement of a lining surface, this may be followed by cancer. So it might well be with the lungs.

A last word about smoking: pipes and cigars *if not* inhaled seem reasonably safe. Inhaled, the stronger and more tarry tobacco may be more irritant. Interestingly, cigarette tobacco in Britain and America tends to be different from that used in pipes and cigars and in continental non-virginian cigarettes, and also it burns at an appreciably higher temperature. Both of these factors may make for great or greater toxicity.

Readers who smoke more than five cigarettes a day, please stop (smoking) now.

Soft water

Glasgow, which has a very soft water supply, has the world's highest IHD rate. We now know that people who live all their lives in soft-water areas probably have a higher IHD rate than those who drink hard water. This interesting epidemological fact is probably related to the mineral content of the water and the way this reacts with body chemistry to fur up the arteries, ie there are good scientific reasons for it and it may be wise to stop softening drinking water.

Stress and personality

Various attempts, mostly by Americans, have been made to define the coronary personality, and to relate him to business tycoons. Certainly, highly strung, anxious, competitive, tired, harassed, unfit, overweight, sedentary people come into this class. Many of them are also successful.

Stress will be discussed in more detail in a later chapter, but it cannot be denied, and support comes from one's own personal social experience, that certain types of people are more likely to get a coronary than others. Similarly, a number of over-conscientious, fussy, pedantic people (company secretaries, for instance) tend also to get coronaries but for slightly different reasons.

These personality factors are to a degree reflected in the individual's body chemistry and his way of life. Indeed, they are inseparable from both. Why, for instance, does one person smoke and not another, and the same goes for weight, exercise, holidays, relaxation and so on. Without going into detail, it is fair to claim that over-tired, overworked, stressed people are, for a variety of reasons, likely to be more coronary prone. Of course, they are also equally more likely to get other diseases. Indeed indigestion and duodenal ulcer is a much less lethal defence mechanism than IHD, but that too is another story.

Miscellaneous factors

There are a number of other factors that contribute to coronary proneness. These are high blood pressure (see Chapter 4), gout (because the uric acid damages the kidneys and puts up blood pressure), other kinds of kidney disease and hormones. In this case, the latter are mostly the steroid sex hormones, which are chemically related to cholesterol.

Eunuchs apparently do not, or perhaps did not, get coronary thrombosis and mostly neither do women until at least ten years after the menopause (change of life). The pill, for instance, tends to put up cholesterol levels. So far there is not much real evidence that it causes coronaries but it may cause thrombosis of other vessels.

The cardiovascular balance sheet

I have devoted a lot of space to describing coronary risk factors, because IHD is the biggest single health hazard facing middle-aged men. If the risks are understood and appreciated they can, it seems, be minimized by appropriate avoiding action. If an individual who is 'at risk' wants to continue on a self-destructive course, this is his affair, although it may be unfair on his company and family. Equally companies, as employers and creators of environments, have a responsibility not to drive their staff by interpersonal and other demands into the high-risk factor group.

In The Medical Centre, one of the things we try to do when every patient has been seen and fully investigated, is to draw up a cardiovascular balance sheet. This involves looking at all the risk factors described, assessing personality, the pressures from work and home, and then throwing in relaxational pursuits and outside interests. One or two not very serious 'below the line' features do not usually matter, unless the man starts in a high-risk category, in which case they probably need dealing with. Three 'bad marks' means urgent avoiding action and so on.

Another important point, which will be discussed later, is that the early manifestations of these 'black marks' produce no symptoms, so that they can only be detected by routine screening as in a health check.

We have done enough of this work to know now that over one-third of the people who come to us have 'black marks' and many of these are alarmingly young, ie under 40. Left alone, they are likely to be in the coronary group. If they get the message and reform, and often this can be quite painful, we think that they are significantly more likely to survive, although we cannot yet prove this.

Figure 2:13 shows, in one group studied, how three risk factors — hypertension, smoking and cholesterol — interact to increase the risk. A man

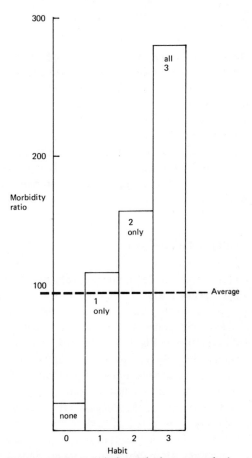

Figure 2:13 Coronary risk factor analysis: effects of one, two, or three risk factors on morbidity ratio (hypertension, smoking, high cholesterol). (Source: Framlingham Community Survey)

with three risk factors has nearly three times the coronary rate. Equally a man with only one is worse off than the fit man against whom there are no black marks.

THREE

Hypertension

Strictly speaking raised blood pressure is a different clinical entity from coronary thrombosis and coronary or cardiac ischaemia (reduced blood supply to the heart muscle), although the heart is obviously and inevitably involved in the blood pressure story as it motivates blood circulation.

We saw in Chapter 2 that in benign hypertension the heart starts working at a higher pressure either because something goes inherently wrong with its control mechanism or because there is an increased demand from perhaps the narrowing and hardening of the arteries, either as a generalized change or a local one related, say, to kidney disease. In either case, we know that normal arteries respond to pressure increases by hardening and narrowing, thus setting up a vicious circle of demand for pressure increase to keep up the circulation.

We saw that atherosclerosis was a generalized disease related to some extent to lipid metabolism. We also need to know that it is to a degree a natural age change in that, as people get older, the normal wear and tear on the vessels and the expected effects of ageing lead to a degree of atherosclerosis. This can affect any or all the vessels in the body, but usually has most effect on the blood supply to the legs and the brain. Perhaps, because of this change, blood pressure tends to drift gently upwards as age increases. An old medical adage says blood pressure should equal 100 plus your age. This is not bad as a very rough guide, give or take ten per cent.

There has been a tendency on the part of lay people perhaps to think that doctors make too much fuss about blood pressure. Perhaps they do, and even pass their anxiety on to their patetients, who in their turn fuss about their own pressure or that of their spouse. All this probably stems again from the life insurance companies who discovered, many years ago, that people with raised blood pressure were a bad risk for life insurance. This is particularly true for younger people, ie a mildly raised pressure in someone of 35 can be very sinister, whereas a higher pressure in a 65 year old probably does not matter or matters much less.

Measurement of blood pressure

When the heart contracts to expell the blood into the aorta and thence to the other arteries, a relatively large amount of blood is suddenly injected into the aorta. Being elastic, the aorta reacts by expanding somewhat to absorb the volume. The subsequent rebound or contraction then helps to push the blood round the arterial system and back into the veins. In fact, this expansion and rebound goes on all round the larger arteries and produces the pulse beat, which can be seen and felt, particularly at the wrist.

A doctor measures the blood pressure by surrounding an artery, in the arm for convenience, with an inflatable cuff. Blowing this up to a pressure greater than that of the blood in the artery will obviously compress the vessel and halt the blood flow. If one then listens over the artery with a stethoscope, which is only a simple listening device, and lets the air out, it is possible to *hear* when the blood flow starts and to record the pressure at which this happens. This is how blood pressure is recorded.

Because of the elasticity of the system, there are in practice two recordable pressures: the ejection pressure and the flow pressure. The first, which is obviously the higher, is called the systolic pressure and the second the diastolic. Blood pressure is recorded as 150/75, for example, meaning a systolic pressure of 150 and a diastolic of 75 which is reasonably normal in middle age.

Clearly then, it should be possible for these two pressures to vary independently and to an extent they do. In clinical terms, we are more concerned about elevation of the diastolic pressure than the systolic, because it is a more accurate reflection of the work rate of the heart and state of the arteries. If elasticity is good, there will be a significant difference, if poor, they will approximate.

Ranges and variation

Inevitably, there has been a tendency on the part of doctors and patients to look for and expect a *normal blood pressure* but, perhaps surprisingly, this is difficult to define. Obviously, one needs a certain minimum pressure to maintain circulation. If this drops too far as in shock or fainting, there is collapse. To a degree, the upper level does not matter, provided it is not harmfully high. What then is harmful? Here particularly in the middle ranges we are often not sure, because on taking a casual reading for the first time, on someone of say 40, and finding it raised, we do not know what this means in terms of whether this is a stable level or the beginning of disease. If, for instance, the raised pressure remains unchanged three years later, the chances are beginning to look as if it is normal for him. If, on the other hand, the pressure has gone up appreciably, the outlook is less good and the condition ought to be dealt with. In fact, three years is far too long to wait and one needs to check much sooner than this. But in practice there is another consideration, which is that blood pressure is varying all the time, so that a single reading under given conditions should only be taken as a general guide as to what is happening to that person at that time, or how he is reacting to the circumstances of the examination. But, obviously, if the pressure is low, average or raised a meaningful message is received to start the doctor thinking and to create the baseline for future management.

Most people can often feel their heart rate and blood pressure varying. Running up stairs produces an increased demand which is met by a rise in both rate and pressure to speed up the flow. Similarly, emotional states (anger is the most characteristic) put up blood pressure and as part of the general relaxation process, it goes down during sleep and tends to be lower in the morning and higher at the end of the day.

In fact, blood pressure is to a degree a reflection of personality. Aggressive and excitable people have higher pressures than placid people but, as already noted, pressure also goes up with weight, so that fat placid people should be expected to have higher than normal pressure, and they mostly do. There is no doubt too, that some kinds of raised pressure are largely due to emotional conflict and anxiety. If this prolonged, it can start off the hypertension circle.

People vary enormously as to the lability of their blood pressure. In some it remains relatively stable and in others it bounces about all over the place. But the overriding point is that, although it is difficult to define a normal, there is a spectrum in relation to age and build, etc, beyond which one can and should begin to be worried that the heart is doing too much work and the blood vessels are in danger of becoming damaged.

Although one should be chary of giving too much significance to a single raised reading, and this is where life insurance companies may be so unfair, one should regard this as an indication for suspicion and further investigation. I take the clinical view that if a patient's blood pressure is raised by the time I have finished my interview, which can be quite probing, it will also go up at other times during his working or social day, and therefore we need to know more about it, and him.

Treatment

Although one should not fuss unduly about blood pressure, and a lot of people, particularly women, live a long time with raised pressures, it needs to be taken seriously, at least until it has been decided that no action is required. We must do this, particularly in the young, because statistically the outlook is bad, and as we cannot yet separate the high-mortality sheep from the low-mortality goats, the least we can do for our patients is to do our best by treating them as 'sheep'.

This is, now, important, because recent experience has shown not only

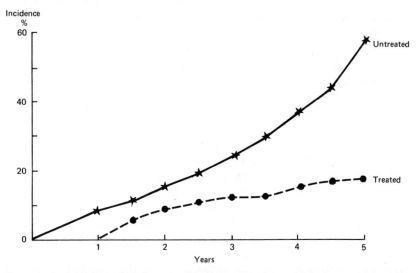

Figure 3:1 Effect of treatment of hypertension on the incidence of strokes, heart and kidney failure. (Source: BUPA Medical Centre)

that with modern drugs, blood pressure is eminently and easily treatable, but also that the results of this treatment are most encouraging in terms of increased life expectancy. The reduction in the incidence of strokes, heart and kidney failure, by treating hypertension, is shown in Figure 3:1.

As obesity is a common disease, it can also be expected to be a common cause of moderately raised blood pressure. Thus, when confronted with an overweight mildly hypertensive patient, the first thing is to get the weight down and then reassess; mostly the weight reduction alone does the trick. If the weight should be normal, it is then necessary to look firstly at the state of the blood vessels, secondly rule out kidney disease and, thirdly, look at the emotional state. Having got all this information plus biochemical and other investigations, one can then decide on the best line of treatment and advice.

If there are strong behavioural or personality characteristics, these may well best be dealt with psychotherapeutically. Sometimes too, small doses of tranquillizers or sedatives are all that is required. Just as with IHD, it may be necessary to try to alter the individual's attitude to his environment, rather than merely treating the symptoms.

As discussed earlier, raised blood pressure damages by overloading the heart which enlarges and then gives up. Also, by encouraging or being associated with arteriosclerosis, blood vessels either burst or block causing a stroke. Coronary thrombosis also occurs as a result of hypertension and is, indeed, one of the end results of this condition. But, in the clinical entity of IHD, as described in Chapter 2, hypertension is only one of the many factors that contribute. A high proportion of people having coronary thrombosis are probably normotensive.

Like IHD then, benign hypertension is a spectrum or progression of pressures which vary from moment to moment from person to person, but there is usually a drift upwards, partly from age and partly as the undesirable result of disease — a disease we do not yet entirely understand. But we do know that the trend upwards tends to be progressive and as it can now be halted, it behoves us, as doctors, to do the best we can to detect early elevations, keep them under observation and intervene if necessary. At The Medical Centre, we feel that many doctors are still too reluctant to intervene and wait to do so until the levels are too high. We call them 'the come back when you are dead' school of doctoring and regard them as people to be avoided by patients. In fact, the climate is changing and there is now a greater willingness to treat early raised blood pressure, particularly in younger people.

Malignant hypertension

In addition to the common benign hypertension, there is a much more sinister, rapidly developing condition, known as malignant hypertension. In this, the blood pressure races away out of control and all the symptoms we have described occur, but much more dramatically. A variant of this condition can occur in women in late pregnancy and, although only over a short term, it can damage the heart vessels or kidneys permanently. Caught early, and unlike benign hypertension it usually produces symptoms, malignant hypertension can be controlled. It is no longer necessarily a death warrant.

For good reasons, conscientious doctors interested in preventive medicine must fuss a bit about blood pressure, but the results of so doing are increasingly encouraging. Equally, people, particularly if they are older, live for many years without a great deal of disability, with surprisingly high pressures. But because of the overriding figures given at the beginning of this section, raised blood pressure must be taken seriously.

Associated complaints

Quite reasonably, because they care about their health and because of the emotional connotation of the heart, and heart disease, people tend to focus attention on their hearts. Lying awake at night, perhaps worrying about something, it is often difficult not to be aware of one's heart beating, and having started on this tack, one may realize that it is not entirely regular. This sensation of the heart beating is called palpitation and it can be very difficult to get away from. I have found in myself that it is often a fatigue symptom, and that it only bothers me when I am overtired.

It can be much worse when the heart is enlarged from hypertension or other disease and this becomes something that the patient has to live with. Similarly, people get into the habit of noticing the heart rate and there are conditions in which the heart suddenly takes off and races away. This is called tachycardia and can, if persistent, be treated. The first patient I saw, who had artificial heart valves inserted, said that particularly if he got up in the night, he could hear his heart change gear and go off at a higher rate to get him down the corridor.

Because anginal pain is a well-known associate of IHD, anxiety tends to give rise to heart and chest pain. Unless there is ischaemia or other heart disease, this pain is nearly always a manifestation of tension and not coronary insufficiency. The pain of the latter too is almost always associated with physical activity whereas the former comes on with reflection. Pain over the heart can also come from the ribs and associated muscles.

The stomach being just below the heart, can if it fills up with wind, press on the diaphragm and displace the heart or slightly interfere with its action. This interference, often worse at night or after meals, frequently gives way after a good burp, but it can cause cardiac anxiety. However, one should be careful never to reassure a patient about cardiac pain without doing a thorough examination including a cardiograph.

FOUR
Other Common Conditions

The biggest and most justified criticism levelled at doctors is that they 'won't tell'. It has always seemed sad that part of the traditional doctor's image of himself as a little tin god is an unwillingness to tell patients about themselves. I feel very strongly that individuals do have a basic right to know what is wrong with them and that the medical services have no right to either withhold this information or replace it with half truths. The fact that the individual may neither like nor understand the true information, is an inadequate general reason for not giving it to them.

Over the last ten years, we have found at The Medical Centre, that the best way of motivating people to change their life styles is to give them the facts and figures, rather as presented so far in this book. Where there are good reasons for a particular course of action, this should be explained and, if there are genuine alternatives, they should be discussed. Businessmen are very well aware that there is often more than one option and they are used to taking calculated risks, but they like either to calculate the odds themselves or at least be privy to the computation. They do not easily accept unsupported statements.

Furthering this philosophy, it seemed that it might be useful to include a little basic information about some of the conditions common in middle age. This is not intended to be complete or exhaustive, but the following pages are aimed at helping your understanding of these conditions. If you know already, or do not want to know any more, press on to the next chapter.

Cancer

All that I have said so far about reticence and traditional medical attitudes comes to a head over cancer. Because it is believed so often to lead to untreatable and uncomfortable death, it is, with dying, the great unmentionable subject in our community at the present time, it being assumed that people do not want to know that they have got cancer. Often this is probably true less than the doctors think, but the 'customer' should at least be given the option rather than have it decided for him.

This attitude is compounded by another tradition in hospitals, that of using a whole series of hopefully misleading euphemisms for the dreaded word, to aid medical discussion and bamboozle the sufferer. All this, of course, helps to perpetuate what I believe to be an unsatisfactory state of affairs. Readers in this situation who are either in doubt or feeling that they are being misled, should fix their informers with a steely eye, stand by for a possible shock and ask the direct question: 'Is it cancer doctor?'

Sometimes the answer may legitimately be 'I don't yet know'. Further tests or a microscopic examination following a small operation called a biopsy may be necessary to reach finality, but go on asking the question. Remember too that in serious conditions affecting life and health, you are always entitled to a second opinion and no good doctor (GP or specialist) should resent this.

Although also being a sign of the zodiac, cancer comes from the Latin — the crab, so called because it creeps through the tissues. But not all cancers creep, some grow slowly and only locally and some, the benign ones, press on local tissues, without invading them. They can usually and easily be shelled out by a surgeon.

Nearly all the cells of the body are in a constant state of cyclical growth, activity and replacement. This is particularly true of the skin and membranes lining the gut. It is also a natural part of healing — how else can 'breaches in the walls' be repaired? All this regenerative growth is under complicated control to keep it orderly and coordinated.

When controls break down groups of cells go berserk locally and reproduce themselves at the expense of their neighbours. Such new growth activity is called cancerous. But not all such new growths are technically cancers — they do not spread by invasion. We all have moles, lumps, bumps and swellings of various sorts and most of these represent a local cellular over-growth. Usually these are benign and only cause a local nuisance. Any cell in the body can behave like this and cause cancer. Invasive tumours (swellings) happen when the growing cells break out and invade or permeate the surrounding tissues. This is a malignant tumour, spread in a variety of possible ways; by local invasion as just described, by getting into the blood or lymphatic system and being carried to a distance where the cells go on growing and produce secondary cancer.

The malignancy of a cancer is determined by a lot of complicated factors: the basic activity of the cell, the age of the patient and the resistance of the host tissues. Tumours in young people tend to be more malignant than tumours in older people. But more older people tend to have cancer as the control mechanisms break down and it is easier for groups of cells to go berserk and lead their own life. In addition to all this, certain chemicals are carcinogenic to certain cell types, ie these chemicals are likely to induce cancer, like aniline dye does in the bladder and several other industrially used chemicals in the nose, lung and skin, etc.

The treatability of cancer depends on a number of factors, as follows. *How accessible it is,* ie swellings or ulcers on the skin, in the mouth, for example are discovered early. *How accessible to treatment* it is, ie can it be easily removed or 'hit' with x-rays without too much other local damage? *How malignant* or rapidly growing it is, whether or not it has invaded and if so how far has it gone, and finally whether or not it is inherently sensitive or treatable in some way, or is it sensitive to radiation or chemicals. Sadly, not all of them are.

Unfortunately, socially we tend to hear only about the cancers for which there is no cure; medicine and cancers general reputation get no credit for the at least equally large number that are successfully treated and forgotten about.

In dealing with cancer, it is essential to realize two things. Firstly, that the chances of cure are vastly greater if diagnosed and treated early. For instance, in breast cancer, the commonest cancer in women, if surgery is performed before the growth has left the breast, a stage 1 case, the survival rate is about 85 per cent, ie there is an 85 per cent chance of a five year cure; but in a stage II case, in which there has been spread, the survival rate drops to less than 30 per cent. Secondly, and especially in older people, all suspicious swellings, symptoms, or bleedings should be reported and investigated. *The cure of cancer thus starts with the individual and not the doctor.*

Figures 4:1 and 4:2 give the incidence and mortality rate from cancers in caucasian men and women. Interestingly, other races and environments produce or have different cancers. Although cancer causes about a third of all deaths, the amount of death caused by an individual type of cancer, say, lung cancer in men, is relatively small, particularly when compared with IHD or hypertension.

Common cancers in men arise from the prostate, lung and stomach and in women, the breast and stomach are the commonest sites.

The future of our battle with cancer, as we are finding in our special women's cancer screening unit, lies in early diagnosis. Just as women themselves forced the ministry to provide facilities for cervical cytology, they should now demand breast screening. Breast cancer is four times as common as cervical cancer. But the main objective is to stop brushing cancer under the carpet and to discuss it and the associated problems openly. The Americans are far better at this than we are. Many years ago I went to the air terminal to meet some American cousins of my wife. They wanted to revisit Scotland before they died. I expected them to be fragile and decrepit, but before we got home in the car, I found the 'he' had had his larynx removed and that

Type of cancer	1941	1951	1961	1971
Lung	230	550	869	1 060
Stomach and pancreas	491	464	453	421
Colon and rectum	463	374	294	304
Prostate	127	143	164	170
Bladder	70	85	96	116
All cancers	1 992	2 120	2 386	2 656
All causes of death	15 692	13 384	12 565	12 157

Figure 4:1 Death rates per million, males of all ages, from cancers. (Source: Registrar General's figures for England and Wales)

Type of cancer	1941	1951	1961	1971
Breast	323	352	389	446
Colon and rectum	363	346	329	341
Stomach and pancreas	315	346	340	303
Lung	48	91	139	224
Womb	210	178	165	153
All cancers	1 681	1 822	1 940	2 147
All causes of death	11 810	11 765	11 376	11 114

Figure 4:2 Death rates per million, females of all ages, from cancers. (Source: Registrar General's figures for England and Wales)

'she' had lost both breasts, her ovaries and pituitary in an effort to control her breast cancer. Their cheerfulness and objectivity has always stuck in my mind.

Respiratory disease: bronchitis, asthma and emphysema

Chronic bronchitis, the English disease, results from local and general air pollution. Cigarette smoking apart (and this makes a bad situation worse), it is a regionally and socio-economically based disease, ie more prevalent in towns and in social classes IV and V.

Pollutional irritation stimulates the lining of the lungs which produce sticky mucus, coughed up as phlegm. Infection grows in the mucus which increases the damage. Thus the whole situation tends to be progressive, with gradual destruction of lung tissue, increasing breathlessness and so on. Small regular doses of antibiotics all through the winter help to control the infection and halt the process. So, of course, does reducing the pollution, like stopping inhaling tobacco smoke.

Asthma is an allergic/stress condition, which often starts in childhood. Perhaps it is more the parents' fault. In it the bronchi, tubes taking air to the lung, go into spasm so that air cannot get in and out. Attacks are usually short, often at night, but do lead, as does bronchitis, to the lungs becoming 'hollow' so that there is not enough tissue left for air exchange. This is called emphysema.

Asthmatics and bronchitics tend to become progressively more crippled as their lungs get destroyed and cannot provide enough oxygen to meet the demands of activity. Their damaged lungs are also very prone to pneumonia and other infection and, indeed, they tend finally to die prematurely, from either this or heart failure.

To a degree, bronchitis is a preventable disease and, although it cannot be cured, it can be held more or less static, largely by removing the irritation. Interestingly, cigarette-smoking businessmen, because of their more favourable environment, have far better lung function than would be expected if they were factory workers. But this is still no excuse for smoking.

Diabetes

Is a disease, one usually milder form of which tends to develop later in life, in which the body's ability to deal with sugar, and hence carbohydrate foods that are converted to sugar during digestion, is impaired. The impairment relates to the production by special cells in the pancreas, of a hormone called insulin. Either too little is produced or it does not work properly for other reasons.

Diabetes is diagnosed mostly by finding sugar in the urine. This happens because the sugar level, blood sugar, goes up above the threshold that the kidney normally holds back. Sugar always circulates in the blood to provide energy and the level, not surprisingly, goes up after meals or eating sweets. Finding sugar in the urine does not necessarily mean diabetes because there may be an unimportant kidney leak. The diagnosis is confirmed by measuring the level in the blood and then by serial measurements every 15 minutes, monitoring how a loading dose of glucose is dealt with. This is known as a glucose tolerance test.

Very mild diabetes is treated by getting the patient's weight down and reducing carbohydrates in the diet. If this does not work, various tablets can be taken and, if this fails, regular daily insulin injections deal with the situation. But a high proportion of older people now manage on tablets alone. Diabetes is important because sufferers tend to wear out prematurely. Infections are more common as is cardiovascular disease, nerve damage and disturbance of vision.

Unexpected and often quite severe diabetes is one of the commoner conditions found at screening examinations. But although it cannot be cured, it can be made very little of a hardship by an intelligent and well-instructed patient. Life insurance companies will often take on all but the most severe diabetics, once they have been controlled.

Blindness: glaucoma and cataract

The inside of the eye, having no blood vessels, is nourished by tissue fluid diffusing through it. There is thus a circulation and drainage system. If this latter gets blocked, pressure builds up in the eye and the visual apparatus is damaged. Early diagnosis and treatment either by drops or drilling 'drain holes' is essential if vision is to be preserved. Glaucoma is said to be the commonest cause of blindness in older people and it tends to run in families. However, it is not common in The Medical Centre practice, although we do test for it in high risk people.

Cataract is a gradually developing opacity in the lens of the eye, which obviously interrupts vision. When it is 'ripe', ie will shell out easily, it can be very satisfactorily dealt with surgically. There are also some new operations using lens transplants which sometimes give good results. Cataract is commoner in diabetes and both this disease and raised blood pressure can also reduce visual acuity by damage to the retina.

It is well known that focusing power in the eye diminishes with age, and regular eye testing is essential about every two years for everyone over 45.

Backache and prolapsed disc

The effective relief of pain in the back is one of the black areas of medicine. In no other, except possibly the related field of rheumatism, is there such a plethora of occasionally . effective treatments. Most of these, like spinal jackets, corsets, traction, special beds, always seem to me to be worse than the disease and often, like corsets, positively harmful, as they encourage the muscles to become weak and lazy.

Back pain is the price of walking upright and holding the head high, while retaining the ability do do up one's shoes and cut one's toe nails, to say nothing of lifting and pushing. To keep the head in the air, the spine has to be strong, and to do all the other things required, it has to be mobile. To manage all this, it has finished up structurally unsound, especially in tall people whose backs are more mechanically vulnerable.

Any or all of the bones, joints, ligaments and associated muscles in the back, can cause back pain. Injury or wear and tear causes arthritis which is an obvious, if difficult to treat, cause of pain.

The bodies of the vertebrae are both held together and allowed to move by elastic intervertebral discs. These have a tough peripheral binding to the bone above and below and a softer elastic central core. They are, in fact, 'elastic washers'. If part of the binding gives way, the core protrudes and should this impinge on say, a nerve, the latter will be irritated and painful down its length. In fact, the nerves are vulnerable to pressure where they emerge from the spinal cord, hence the condition known as sciatica.

Prolapsed disc pain can come and go, but if there is overt nerve damage, operation is often advisable and now usually effective.

But much back pain, particularly in women, has no obvious cause and tends not to respond to treatment. Perhaps the back becomes the dumping ground for life's discontents. Similarly, muscle tension, a reflection of general tension, can also cause pain.

A vulnerable back can be very limiting. Any treatment which helps, is to my mind legitimate and osteopaths tend to be better at manipulating than many doctors. Quite often, manipulation seems to relieve spasm and symptoms. In my view, it is desirable, firstly, to do everything possible to maintain muscle strength and, secondly, to think very seriously before being incarcerated in bed or plaster for long periods.

Cervical discs and arthritis in the neck is now a popular disease. It causes local pain and tingling which also radiates down the arms to the fingers. This can be worse at night.

Arthritis and rheumatism

Arthritis is a wear and tear condition of joints which creak and are painful like a rusty hinge. It is either an age change or follows earlier injury. Hips are particularly prone and can now be dealt with well by surgery. Thus, individuals who played violent games when young or had other joint injuries are more likely to get arthritis in middle age.

Rheumatism (and fibrositis) is one of the blanket words which, hopefully, means something to the patient while concealing the doctor's almost complete ignorance of what the pain is due to. The term is applied to generalized muscular pain which may also be provoked by nerve irritation or come directly from bones, joint and ligaments. General muscular and body tension causes quite a lot of it and muscles can be felt in spasm, but basically little is known about either cause or treatment, except that massage, heat, aspirin, copper bracelets and a host of other remedies sometimes effect cures.

Rheumatoid arthritis is quite a different, but well-defined condition (different from both rheumatism and the wear and tear osteoarthritis). It is an inflammatory condition of the smaller joints mostly. Hands, wrists and elbows are the most commonly involved. There is intense pain, swelling and general misery, followed by considerable deformity and loss of function.

Little is known about the cause of this relatively common disease. It is seen more often in women, many of whom are obviously unhappy. In my view, too little attention has been paid to the psychological aspects of rheumatoid arthritis.

Treatment is aimed at controlling pain and inflammation, and minimizing deformity. At a later stage surgery may be required to deal with the deformity. Anti-inflammatory drugs include aspirin and its derivatives, Indocid, Butazolidine and steroids. Injections of gold and other substances are also used. Most of the drugs, including aspirin, have potentially dangerous side effects.

Until the cause is known and understood, treatment is unlikely to become more effective. Rheumatologists are an odd lot who have a thankless task grappling with conditions they do not understand and can seldom cure. Because of this, they have a very restrictive and 'keep off the grass' attitude to non-doctors who offer, often neither more nor less successfully, alternative treatments. I am very much in favour of osteopaths.

Indigestion: peptic ulcer, hiatus hernia and bowel trouble

Indigestion, often intermittently chronic, is a seldom lethal but relatively common group of conditions. The digestive tract starts in the mouth and ends at the anus. Pain can arise from any part of the gullet (oesophagus) stomach, duodenum, small or large intestine. The smooth or not so smooth coordination of the digestive system is often a reflection of general well-being. But malfunction can also be related to indiscretion, fatigue or anxiety.

The stomach is a reservoir which produces acid to start off digestion. It has to be tough to deal with the acid, but the constant insult and irritation of 'strong foods' like curry, and alcohol, cause it to be inflamed and irritable — known as gastritis — resulting in nausea, vomiting and diarrhoea.

The duodenum is the first part of the small intestine and gets the full blast of the acid stomach contents. But, in spite of this, little is known about why some people get gastric and duodenal ulcers and not others. Ulcers are a common cause of digestive discomfort. The waxing and waning, often with the general life situation, can come to dominate the individual's existence. Like other ulcers, they can bleed and also cause obstruction.

Treatment is by modifying diet and life style, neutralizing acid, reducing smoking and alcohol and, if all this fails, by surgery. There used to be a wide range of diets advised for ulcers, but now it is agreed that peace and quiet and minimal irritation are just as good as milk drips and minced chicken.

The gullet passes through the diaphragm to enter the stomach. There is a muscular 'pinch valve' at its lower end. This stops acid stomach contents getting into and irritating the gullet. Weakness of the diaphragm, which often allows part of the stomach up into the chest, stops the valve functioning. This is called a hiatus hernia. Symptoms are influenced by gravity as when lying down, bending down to tie shoe laces, allows reflux to occur. This causes local burning pain and considerable discomfort. If simple measures like sleeping with the head of the bed raised and on the right side, and alkalis, do not make life bearable, surgery is usually successful.

If the stomach distends with wind, and why it should is mysterious, it presses upwards on the diaphragm and heart and can cause mild chest pain and palpitation, which raises the suspicion of a coronary.

The small intestine causes rather little trouble, but the large one is concerned with constipation, diverticulitis, cancer and generalized inflammatory colitis. Most left-sided abdominal pain in older people tends to be called diverticulitis, as is much other bowel disfunction. In fact, although diverticulae (little out pouches of the bowel), are common, proper inflammation is rare and dangerous as they may perforate.

Constipation and bowel function generally, is an emotive subject. It is best to try and let the digestive tract work and discharge at its own pace. There is no harm from it working slowly, but a surprising number of people fuss if it does.

Bowel disturbance, pain, alteration of habit, bleeding or discharge should be properly investigated, if it does not rapidly recover. Investigations tend to be undignified and uncomfortable and involves the insertion of barium suspension or optical devices on tubes or stalks. Barium being x-ray opaque, outlines the digestive tract and allows abnormalities to be 'profiled'. Cancer of the bowel is mostly eminently treatable. Please report all bleeding to your doctor. Most bleeding comes from piles or ulcers, but all rectal bleeding must be assumed to come from something else until proved otherwise, by looking to see where it comes from.

Gallbladder disease

This is usually in the form of stones, and causes pain, wind and difficulty in dealing with fats, ie fried or fatty foods cause indigestion. Gallstones are often found by chance at screening. Small multiple stones which get dislodged, cause more symptoms than large ones which stay put. Both are probably best removed.

Indigestion is a major reflection of general dis-ease. Indeed dyspepsia is a good description of what the person feels and looks like if he is at odds with his digestion.

But digestive dis-ease, although common, is much less dangerous than using the cardiovascular system as the escape valve. One can say this because dyspepsia provokes symptoms which demand attention whereas IHD is a surprise until it strikes. There being much less to induce avoiding action.

We know that the stomach is to a degree influenced by emotion, as there was a famous case of a Canadian, part of whose stomach came outside following injury. He was studied extensively by physiologists and physicians and a great deal learnt about digestion and indigestion. It is certain, for instance, that sensitive stomachs can blush!

Varicose veins

By starting to walk upright, Man did his back and his veins no good for neither were properly designed to stand the strain.

Back pressure on leg veins with weak valves, which may be hereditary, can cause them to dilate and become varicose. They are then unsightly, particularly in women who do not continually wear trousers, and sometimes but rather idiosyncratically painful. (Varicose veins, for instance, used to be a good way of getting a pension in the army.) They may cause swelling of the ankle and interfere with the nutrition of the skin, giving itching and ulcers. If damaged, they can cause torrential bleeding which stops instantly if the leg is lifted above the heart, by lying down and elevating it.

Varicose veins tend to get worse rather than better with time and should be dealt with, by an expert, by injection or operation.

Haemorrhoids (piles) are varicose veins of the anus. They cause bleeding, discomfort, itching and discharge. Because treatment is undignified and unpleasant it is surprising how many people put up with thoroughly demeaning piles for so long. They should be dealt with by surgery (a thoroughly good operation) or, if small, by injection.

Hernia

Organs, like the testicles in men, have to come out through the abdominal wall. This leaves a potential weak area through which other and unwanted things may later protrude.

A hernia (rupture) is a protrusion of abdominal contents through the wall, usually into the groin. It is locally painful, worse on coughing or straining, as when trying to pass water with an enlarged prostate, and tends to be both uncomfortable and to get bigger. There is also a tendency for the contents to get stuck, causing obstruction, which can be dangerous, and demands emergency surgery.

When surgery and anaesthesia were less competent, there used to be a tendency to hold the rupture back by a steel spring which was a cross between a cork and a chastity belt, called a truss. The present day simple operation is a vast improvement on the wearing of this contraption.

Prostatic enlargement

After about the age of 60, sometimes before, the prostate gland may enlarge benignly. As it surrounds the urethra, which conducts urine from the bladder to the penis, it interferes with emptying the bladder. This may be in terms of urgency, dribbling, difficulty in stopping and starting and inability to totally empty the bladder. Bladder pressure builds up and may damage the kidneys and the residual urine may get infected, which makes the frequency worse.

A particularly troublesome symptom is frequency at night which interferes with sleep. Once it is apparent that prostatic enlargement is causing trouble, the offending gland should be removed. This is now a relatively simple and safe operation, which brings much relief. It should be done early rather than late, at a time to suit the patient and not as an emergency for obstruction, and before it has done damage.

Contrary to folklore, prostatectomy does not stop sexual activity, although it may cause sterility because it may stop ejaculation. But full sexual activity continues.

Talking of sterility, middle-aged men with an adequate family, should seriously consider vasectomy. This is a harmless out-patient or weekend operation which removes all anxiety about other and less effective methods of birth control and again in no way interferes with sexual prowess.

Sex after sixty?

Perfectly normal either way is the short answer to that heading.

Individuals and couples vary with regard to their sexual needs and inclinations as they get older. What they want to go on doing seems to depend on what they have been used to, ie couples who have fairly regular intercourse, say once a week, tend to want to go on. Couples who have much less tend to tail off as they get older.

This can become very much a problem in terms of mutual need and is one for joint discussion. There is no reason why sexual intercourse should not be continued until late in life, but only if it is wanted and enjoyed. Trouble seems to arise when needs vary and one partner is interested and the other not. Unless it is brought out into the open and discussed, this can lead to both friction and guilt about letting the other down. Should it become a serious problem, it should be discussed with a sympathetic expert.

We find, perhaps increasingly, that impotence is a not uncommon problem for men over fifty. Much of it is due to severe and generalized fatigue, leading to sexual disinclination. It appears likely that tiredness is at least as great an enemy to middle aged libido as is alcohol. The critical question here is, does it get better on holiday? Often it does. Sometimes a solution to this type of falling off is to try for intercourse weekend mornings rather than late at night. More serious impotence is for psychological reasons and sometimes these, if mild, can be overcome when young, but get worse with age, fatigue and perhaps marital friction. But failure or relative failure inevitably provokes guilt and anxiety which in turn builds up tension so that performance is further diminished.

Recent impotence replacing previous reasonable or adequate competence should be treatable. Long-standing impotence is much more difficult to deal with. Injections of replacement hormone sometimes helps. But fancy and expensive virilizing injections, sold largely by foreign doctors, have no direct effect, but may give a psychological boost. The money is better spent on a holiday.

Depression

We now know that moderate or severe depression is both common, treatable, frequently missed by doctors and not reported by patients. The depressed person, man or woman, knows that *he is depressed;* he feels gloomy and unable to get stuck into anything. He invents trivial things to do which hopefully make him look busy, but his colleagues and his secretary know that he is not 'decision taking'. Obviously, if he is a senior person, this can be very bad for his company. Depression, of course, also leads to suicide.

A cardinal symptom is alteration of sleep rhythm which contributes to the general disinclination to do anything. The whole situation can, and often does, lead to a considerable increase in alcohol intake. This again points towards the wrong diagnosis, particularly if the person was previously known to be a heavy drinker.

Although the individual knows that he is performing badly and feels perfectly awful, he may be loath to admit it, or if he does all the investigations are normal. The patient is either told to pull himself together or gets sent on a holiday.

A man who was sent on two useless holidays, took to drink and was eased out of his partnership before getting the right treatment, came to see us recently. He was anxious to get senior managers and depressed individuals to realize that this was a treatable condition and that, like alcoholism, it should be dealt with rather than tolerated.

Appropriate treatment, which is not by tranquillizers, but by specific anti-depressants, can be dramatically and rapidly successful. Change of mood, loss of drive, ineffectiveness, coming on to middle age, with or without cause, should be suspected as being due to depression until proved otherwise. Diagnosis may not always be easy, as the spectrum from legitimate gloom, in gloomy people, to suicide is infinitely variable. But suspecting this common condition is the first step to diagnosis.

Alcoholism

The borderline between regular heavy drinking and alcoholism is hard to define. It is very much a drug of addiction, although it is also both a tranquillizer and social lubricant. Apart from becoming a habit, and much of life consists of habits and rituals, it may be the refuge of the weak, the insecure and the unsuccessful. Once someone becomes alcohol dependant, ie cannot easily give it up for several days, and starts drinking well before lunch or supper, he should be regarded as alcoholic. In addition, it is highly likely that his drinking is beginning to interfere with his professional or social competence. In this case, he should certainly be regarded as an alcoholic and made to undergo treatment.

Individuals should watch their drinking as they get older, particularly if they tend to take more than three or four drinks a day. Alcohol is a drug of addiction and overdrinking is a slippery slope down which it is easy to slide gently.

But in reasonable amounts, I am strongly in favour of alcohol as a relaxer, lubricant and pleasure. Remember, however, that it is a high-calorie food and if it is consumed other sources of calories, like bread and potatoes, should be avoided.

Because of the conspiracy of silence about alcoholics in a company or family, there is a reluctance by employers to do anything about it, except in America where large companies all now have overt anti-drug abuse programmes. Wives have little leverage in these cases, they merely suffer and get bruised. The main lever is 'job jeopardy'. Alcoholics need their jobs to maintain their status and self-respect and it is almost only through their employer taking a tough line that they can be goaded into accepting treatment. They should be firmly told that unless they stop drinking and get treated, they will be sacked; if they are ever found incapacitated again, they will have to go, etc. Given a reasonably strong character, this will usually work.

Remember, however that alcoholics are clever and deceitful and seldom admit their habit. They have to be faced with it, with brutal frankness.

One of the least attractive myths of business life is that buying, selling, marketing, advertising and public relations can only be done with alcoholic lubrication. Senior managers have a considerable responsibility to protect their more junior staff from going down the slope. This can easily be done by setting new traditions and watching expense accounts. It will pay handsome dividends in the end, and the customers too might be grateful.

Without making too much of a fetish of it, constant vigilance to see that alcohol consumption does not slowly increase, either individually or in the lunch room, is a wise precaution.

We are often asked, when carrying out a medical examination, if a man is an alcoholic. Although it is a legitimate question to ask, it can be one which is very difficult to answer, because one can only largely go on what the patient says, and a wise alcoholic dries out for a day or two before coming. But alcohol mostly 'hits' the liver which stops functioning efficiently. This loss of function can be shown by special biochemical tests of liver function. Indeed, we often find minor degrees of undesirable change in otherwise fit regular heavy drinkers. This chance finding is nearly always enough to get them to cut down. The liver is mercifully a very adaptive organ and soon recovers.

FIVE

Stress and its Causes

Personality-environment conflict

One of my first patients was sent through my mother, a gynaecologist specializing in family planning. She used to try to insist that all her patients came back about once a year to see that all was well and that no new problems had arisen – good preventive maintenance. In the course of this, she established a most fruitful relationship with her patients as 'wives'. Because of anxiety expressed by one woman about her husband's general state of misery, he was advised to come and see me, 'my son specializes in people like your husband', she said. Little did he realize that at that stage, I would probably learn more from him than vice-versa.

However, once he started talking about himself, it was soon apparent that he was in charge of a large unit in a small chain of building and joinery companies. Unfortunately he was not really in charge because 'ownership' rested in the hands of a series of family trusts, as so often happens, by about the third generation, because of death-duty considerations. Also there was an aged and ineffective chairman who was to a degree manipulated by the family, of which my man was a member, seemingly through his wife.

Clearly there was no effective control or coordination of the group as such, although it was admitted that it was drifting rather than foundering. Subsequently the man, who was around 55 and thoroughly frustrated, listed his personal options. These were, as they always are:

1   To try to organize a revolution presumably to put him into the dominant position.

2   To get out and do something else.

3   To put up with it and stop grumbling, ie an objective decision to accept the status quo counts as *a decision* and if cheerfully accepted should solve or significantly reduce the conflict. A point to which we will return.

As to option-1 he was a bit too feeble to achieve this and, in any case, was not too popular with the family. Had he been born more of a revolutionary he would probably have been the chairman already.

As to 2, what in fact had he to offer on the labour market and who would pay him anything like the salary and perks he was currently getting for being frustrated? So for personality and other reasons he had to stick it out, negotiate an early retirement pension, become a bit more militant as a manager, and then soldier on not too unhappily. All this he did, and providence unexpectedly removed the chairman who was succeeded by a more effective and less outmoded character. This man later doubtless sold the whole group off to some frustrating conglomerate, although they weren't called that in those days.

The reader might ask, what on earth this has got to do with doctoring? I could easily have sent him on a cruise, given him some sleeping pills and tried to boost his libido, which was what was worrying his wife. This might have relieved the symptoms, but I wanted to deal with the causes, which were 'him' and his 'situation' by finding out about all of them.

This, and close association with John Tyzack, the management consultant (we used to exchange 'problem patients' frequently with each other), gave me a fascinating if somewhat frightening insight into the perils of the family firm. Running any company is difficult enough but to try to do this, often with limited talents and no proper training, through a network of scions of the not so noble breed and family trusts, can be, and mostly was, pure hell.

Diverting into anecdotal reminiscence for a minute, I saw another and much more lively man who was chairman and managing director of a very prosperous manufacturing company in the Midlands. He had slightly under a controlling interest and was shattered to find himself suddenly voted out of office at an AGM. This was done not on the grounds that the company was doing badly, because it patently was not, but because they felt he did so many outside things that surely it ought to do better, if only he would devote more time to it.

He knew that really it had more or less reached its potential and also that the man they were putting in was useless. He left the meeting in a state of fury, leapt into a plane and dashed off to Australia, where he knew there were some more cousins with whose shares he could control the company. Having bought these, he waited for a year or so to demonstrate how bad his successor was, then he sold the company and went off and did something quite different.

Tyzack was once trying to reorganize a family concern and thought that he had done this by persuading the 'old man' to become President and let his son 'have a go'. A year or so later, the son sought him out and complained bitterly that Dad was interfering and wrecking the company. When Tyzack went to remonstrate with the old man, the latter said with a twinkle 'it is my company, I made it, and I will wreck it if I want to'.

In another very successful company making a nationally known home product, father, who had 'inherited and improved', despised his slightly wet but not all that bad son. As he had cancer of the prostate and knew he was dying, he turned up at the office one morning and announced to his son and sister, both of whom were directors, that he had sold them out to a larger, food manufacturer.

This type of situation and, indeed, roughly similar ones in bigger and more bureaucratic organizations are worth quoting because they so vividly illustrate a type of stress which arises from the interplay of personality and environment, and also the way in which the 'whole life' of the actors or participants become involved in their stress situation.

Against this background, and at the risk of recovering some of the ground staked out in the introductory chapter, let us now look in a little more detail at the dynamics of this stress situation.

Environment challenge

To recapitulate, we saw that essentially 'stress' was a basic fact controlling life. The survival of Darwin's 'evolutionary fittest' depends on the fitter or more successful members of a plant, animal or fish community overcoming the challenge of the environment better than the rest of the group. This skill, which may have been physical in terms of a slightly larger beak, tongue or claw, or 'intellectual' in being better at exploiting the resources they had is passed on to the next generation and builds up a more successful strain.

All plant and animal life is challenged by the largely physical environment, and it is this challenge that produces the 'dynamic' to keep it going. In humans what is called sensory deprivation, causes disintegration of the personality and behaviour disorder.

If one takes a physically fit and mentally stable individual and puts him or her in an environmentally perfect situation, with optimal heat, ventilation, humidity, food, etc, but in an entirely dark and soundproof room, the subject rapidly becomes uncomfortable. Particularly so, if he or she is made to lie on a comfortably moulded couch, so that postural sensation is minimized. Under these highly artificial conditions, there is virtually no sensory input to keep the subject's nervous system alert. Without any such input to keep it purposefully active, control within the brain breaks down and various parts of it produce random activity. This is reflected in disoriented behaviour, great unease and temporary disintegration of the personality. 'Madness' is much the same phenomenon, but for different reasons. Normal controls and reactions break down and behaviour becomes uncontrolled.

In a different way, of course, solitary confinement can have some of the same effect, and those who have successfully lived through this situation will tell that their survival depended on intense mental discipline with which they kept their bearings. Also, of course, they had the very obvious challenge of the hostile environment to contend with.

The point here is that, in biological terms, challenge from the environment, physical and for humans mostly interpersonal, is essential to keep life going. As far as man is concerned, an additional factor comes in, the relationship between motivation and satisfaction. The reasons why we do things are complicated and range from the personal need (food, sleep, etc), expected cultural and behavioural patterns, need for income; to idiosyncratic personal quirks. But underlying most of this is the joy and satisfaction of succeeding in whatever the activity is.

When we consider any aspect of the 'dilemma of man', it is worth remembering the rapidity of our psycho-social evolution. In terms of learning and experience, we have achieved far too much in not much over 20 000 years, compared with the many thousands of years required for biological evolution. Our present dilemma is that we can alter the environment more quickly than we can adapt to the alterations.

When we begin to consider human behaviour we find that one of the main tone-generating or enlivening functions is to succeed in overcoming challenge or to achieve certain defined goals. On the whole, success is morale boosting and failure morale lowering. Related to overt failure is the parallel situation in which success or progress is prevented by the frustrations and limitations inherent in the system. As in the family firms just mentioned, and most manifestations of the bureaucratic octopus with which we, as tax payers, see fit to surround ourselves, progress or action appears impossible. Frustration becomes a major cause of relative failure and hence of stress.

Defining stress

The difficulty of trying to talk about stress is that it is a misunderstood and, seemingly, misused term. When we say that someone is 'stressed' we mean to imply that life has become too much for him, that he is not making the grade, ie that things are wholly or partly wrong. This may well be the case, but in making and accepting the statement, the sufferer gets no credit for the challenge he has probably withstood before he *became stressed*. Thus, we really require two phrases, one implying challenge overcome, or life adequately dealt with, and the other implying as stress now does, defeat or relative defeat; but it is unfair to consider only one aspect of the situation.

Stress is a term taken by biology from engineering, where it is in fact better used. In engineering, stress implies an inherent capacity to withstand strain. Inert structures like steel girders or timber joists have a calculable strength and an inherent strain or distortion resistance related to their shape, size and the material they are made of. If, however, overloading occurs, the structure will distort and fracture but perhaps surprisingly, if in this respect the word stress is used at all, it is qualified as the . . . . . . was overstressed. Technology has now taken this even further. The strength, or strain resistance of some structures can be considerably enhanced by what is called prestressing, the biological equivalent of which is possibly adaptation.

Thus, it appears that the word stress is correctly used in engineering but becomes inadequate when applied to people. However, as no-one has so far been able to produce an alternative term, we shall have to stick to 'stress' as implying that the individual or group referred to is, or might soon be, overloaded. Hopefully, it will always be remembered that, depending on the person's threshold, a good deal of activity, conflict or challenge must have been dealt with previously to produce this stressed situation.

Assessment of stress

When we were clinically groping our early way towards a better understanding of the role of stress in dis-ease and what this did to people, we very soon found that in trying to evaluate executives in business or domestic situations, it was wise to first try to make some assessment of the stress or forces involved. Mostly this had to be done as a quality judgement based on inadequate and perhaps one-sided evidence, but in terms of coming to a useful stress summary, we first tried to decide how stressful the situation was, at work or at home, and then, as the second stage, to decide how well or badly the individual was coping.

This is in practice an important distinction because, particularly in terms of the executive environment, a man got better marks for standing up well to what was by any standards a tough situation, than did one who was making a fuss, and hence failing, at a much lower level of strain. In both cases one was primarily concerned to help the individual deal with his problems, but because the breaking point was so different, one was likely to be dealing with problems at two different levels of complexity.

Work situations like this were made more fascinating and easier to deal with if one doctor dealt with the whole executive group. Clearly his first responsibility, and the main object of the exercise, was to assess and help the individual. Working along these lines, every member of the group seen added to the doctor's picture of the situation and his assessment of the climate within the company. Soon, if he is perceptive, he begins to realize what they are doing to each other, good and bad, and how this might affect the well-being of the company as a whole. As experience developed we began to be in a position to be able to advise companies, at least those who wanted to know, about what their interpersonal or psycho-social climate was like.

Business too, for obvious reasons, tends to attract dominant people, but many of them completely fail to understand the effect of their behaviour on those below them. As we were tough, independent and concerned, we could and often did, if our terms of reference were right, take the chairman aside, for instance, and tell him some of the things about himself which he ought to have known ages ago, but which his staff were too frightened to bring up. By so doing, with a few home truths, and perhaps throwing in some points on working conditions, like holiday or travel rules, hours of work, etc., one could sometimes quite dramatically alter the climate within the organization, hopefully for the better. This became useful and fascinating preventive medicine.

I was once a regular speaker at one of the management training colleges and they asked me to see a student who seemed to be on the verge of a breakdown. This man was the works manager of a small unit in a large diversified company. He had been promoted to set up and commission a new factory in a rather remote, previously non-industrial area. As usually happens in these situations, nothing went right and everyone got rather tired and frayed. In the end, and a bit late, it all worked out well and the unit was established and productive but our man remained tired, irritable and doubtless was a bit short with everyone.

One day there was a knock on his door and his welfare supervisor came in, very timid and frightened. She said, 'Look Mr X, I am sorry, but I must come and talk to you.' 'Do you realise', she asked 'what effect it has on the staff of this factory, every time you lose your temper with someone?' and she went on to spell this out in more detail.

The man was grateful and took it to heart, but someone above him had also spotted that he was under too much strain and, instead of doing the sensible thing and sending him on a holiday, he was sent on a middle management training course. Here, he felt even more inadequate, was overcome by remorse about the awful things he had done to the people under him and when I saw him he was on the verge of an anxiety breakdown.

Reactions to stress

We must now return to the dynamics of the basic stress/strain situation and explore what might happen when 'stress' becomes potentially harmful. If challenge from the environment is part of the biological life, it is likely that defence mechanisms will have been developed to protect the organism from 'over challenge'. In fact this is what has occurred and the defense reactions are just as much a part of normal behaviour as the need for challenge.

Thus for humans, when a situation becomes too much for them, there has to be a formula under which they can disengage without loss of esteem, or damage. If the strain on an individual becomes unbearable, he becomes stressed and develops a *stress reaction*. This is designed to take him temporarily out of the firing line. In practice, he becomes dis-eased and tends to develop symptoms or an abnormality of behaviour, designed biologically, as it were, to shunt him sideways and get him off the hook. Pain in one form or another is, of course, the commonest symptom.

Unfortunately, this explanation is both over simplified and too mechanistic because most of the chain of cause and effect is not consciously realized and the individual is seldom aware of what is happening. All he knows is that he has a splitting headache, roaring indigestion, insomnia or whatever. This is because the reaction is automatic and essentially occurs at an unconscious or subconscious level. As learning proceeds from birth onwards, the simple reactions get overlaid in all sorts of ways by personality quirks and learned behaviour reactions.

When I was a medical student all symptoms which had no discernable organic basis, that is a detectable change in the tissues or blood biochemistry, were called functional or neurotic. They were regarded as weakness of the moral fibre and rather written off, largely because they were not then understood at all. Now we realize that behavioural symptoms are just as real and significant as organic ones and that both represent a call for help from a dis-eased person, ie an acute anxiety state is just as real an illness as acute appendicitis.

Psychologists from Freud onwards have taught us how infinitely complicated our seemingly simple behaviour may be. In life we practically never respond in a simple, natural and basic way.

In practice, how we react to a given situation, at any age, is determined by our personality, intelligence and temperament, etc, and our past experience. Growing up, too, consists of acquiring a whole chain of learned responses. Society expects certain reactions and behaviour patterns. Not only do these have to be learnt, but often other more simple and natural ones have to be supressed or inhibited. For instance, in basic biological terms, excretion is a necessary natural function, as is sexual activity, but both have become so overloaded with 'expected behaviour' that the real reaction gets driven underground. Even to the extent of producing guilt reactions in children and adults.

The same type of thing happens, particularly in childhood, in relation to basic emotional needs. Bad handling of a child by either or both parents can completely alter its behaviour; deprivation of basic emotional need and support has a similar effect. The difficulty is that the learned and usually defensive response which, as it were, buries both the deprivation and the natural response, puts up a wall between the individual and the world, behind which he shelters. So also does the possible development of a parallel series of responses to compensate for emotional or other deprivation or inadequacy.

In this way, layers of experience get overlaid with layers of expected and protective reactions. When seen years later, in a middle-aged adult, as a certain and perhaps harmful or personality-limiting behaviour pattern, it is difficult to unscramble the chain of cause and effect of what is now being defended against.

As well as this group of 'happenings' individuals have, or should have, a series of basic drives or needs which they have to learn to requite and deal with in accordance with opportunity, personality and social mores. In this way, the adult personality develops. All individuals have attributes related to genetic inheritance, upbringing and what they have made of their previous experience.

To give one rather simple example, if a somewhat introverted child has parents who expect too much of it and are always running the child down, and making both their disappointment in the child's incompetence quite clear, it would have to be a very tough child indeed to survive becoming an insecure and inferior feeling person. It would also find adult relationships with its parents difficult because of the earlier denigration.

The point about the role of a defence mechanism is two-fold. Firstly, it can take any one of an almost infinite range of reactions. Secondly, the reaction will probably not be perceived by the individual as in any way defensive. All he will say is, 'hell, I've got my headache again' or 'I feel absolutely rotten and must go home'. In clinical practice, at least up to a few years ago, it was surprising how few reasonably intelligent people were ever prompted into working out what produced quite significant symptoms like migraine or severe dyspepsia. If one could establish a chain of cause and effect for a set of symptoms, which could then be explained to the sufferer, the symptoms could then be regarded as a warning that something is going wrong. 'Get to know your devil', was my advice, and he will become a friendly devil who will help to keep you out of worse trouble. The onset of symptoms can thus be used as a warning that margins were narrow.

The defence mechanism, when life, either consciously or unconsciously becomes too much, causes the 'patient' to gradually opt out. If he realizes in time what is happening, he may just decide that it is time to stop and take a break, otherwise something will go wrong with his mechanisms and he will become dis-eased in some way, which will protect him from further exposure.

Range of reactions and thresholds

What we call disease is a spectrum of disability, some of it caused by outside or infective or toxic agents, some of it appears to result from, or cause the malfunctioning of, a body mechanism, as in a peptic ulcer or headache, and some is a straight behaviour disturbance such as insomnia, irritability or anxiety, etc. Two more points may be made in relation to this concept. The first is that the range of possible reactions is almost infinite and theoretically it does not matter whether the dis-ease takes an organic or behavioural form. It is increasingly being believed that most of all disease is psychosomatic in origin, ie that it represents a primarily or initially defensive reaction by the individual against the demands of the environment.

In medical terms this is a difficult concept to justify. We know that the tubercle bacillus causes pulmonary tuberculosis and that the typhoid bacillus causes typhoid, but it is not known why, if 100 people are exposed to either, only a few of them will be infected. In addition, we do not know why one person will respond to pathological or harmful stress by getting a peptic ulcer, another a coronary and the third say a skin rash. We are beginning to know some of the ways in which certain types of people may characteristically react. It is apparent that to a degree the reaction will depend on basic personality, perhaps body build and also inevitably on past experience. Thus, children whose mother had migraine or asthma or bilious attacks tend to 'inherit' this as a shared environmental factor and to adopt it as 'their disease'; it becomes the family reaction. 'We all had weak tummies', for example.

The second and very important point is that individuals have differing thresholds to seemingly similar stress situations. Some are born tougher than others and will survive better or longer. As we all know, the world is sadly full of inadequate people who just do not seem to be able to cope with life at all. They have a very low stress threshold and fold up easily. Because they tend to be made of 'straw', it is not really much help merely knowing what their stresses are and what motivates their reactions. Unhappily, it is seldom possible to put backbone back into them, but sometimes one can do a little. Unfortunately, understanding stress and using it as a philosophical framework to explain health and disease is not a magic key which opens all doors to successful cure, and psychotherapy cannot cure all behaviour disturbance.

Another fundamental point is that any one individual is likely to have varying abilities to deal with or stand up to different types of demand or challenge. Thus, one person may be good at dealing with things in a technical way and thoroughly bad at dealing with people. Another might be good at people in the office, but bad with his family at home. The way in which these challenges are dealt with, will both reflect his personality and determine his skill in dealing with life. If, however, the limitations are realized and understood, the 'weakness' can at least be diminished if not made into a positive strength. Admitting faults is in practice a virtue as necessary as assessing oneself objectively.

The variability of these thresholds has important implications for both professional and domestic life. They mean that no two people will react in the same way or break down simultaneously. I may work well with A and you with B. Swap either of us or A and B and there may well be tension leading to chaos. Thus in industry and commerce, as in life, the importance of 'horses for courses' must never be lost sight of. One of the skills of management is to manipulate the environment so as to get the best out of, and minimize the friction on, the human resource available to it.

The other important thing is that many dis-ease (defense) patterns get built in as part of life and their sudden removal can be disastrous, ie the treatment may be worse than the disease. One man who came to see me, walked in, looked me over and announced firmly that he had had severe indigestion ever since his mother died 20 years ago. My spontaneous and tactless reaction, was to say, 'Good God haven't you got over that yet?'. This rather callous and unsympathetic response to his usual call for help destroyed a useful relationship. Without any warning I had pulled out the prop on which he had been trading for years, but I did cure his indigestion.

Another good case, illustrative of how these responses can work, refers to a 14 year-old girl who fairly suddenly developed serious asthma, so serious was it that the ordinary remedies did not control the spasms and recourse was being had to undesirably large doses of steroids.

Luckily, the child soon fell into the hands of a very perceptive psychiatrist who 'discovered' that the girl, being bright, had won a grammar-school place. She also had a very ambitious mother who was determined that her daughter should do well. Unfortunately, however, the girl herself did not like this at all but wanted to go to the local secondary modern school and stay with her friends. By getting asthma she not only avoided the hated school, but also kept her mother home from work to look after her. Once all this had been sorted out and explained, there was no need for steroids. If it had not been dealt with, the child would probably have become a life-long asthmatic and fifteen years later only psychoanalysis might have discovered why.

Causally related reactions

One last point about the mind and body philosophy of illness is that we are slowly learning more about the possible mechanisms of the interrelations of body control systems to produce some of the changes that constitute disease. That emotional states can cause physical change has been apparent for as long as humans observed each other. Laughing, crying, blushing, etc, are all physical expressions of emotion. In much the same way grief can effect the way in which the 'whole person' reacts and similarly anxiety or tension can upset basic body functions like the bowels and the bladder and perhaps most important of all, sleep.

If these relatively simple reactions are causally related, it is not unlikely that other more complicated ones can be similarly provoked. All the body's systems and reactions are coordinated and controlled chemically and/or through the nervous system. To a degree at any rate, this controls the 'body tone' which can in turn effect reactions like immunity and resistance to disease, as well at the extent to which groups of cells break lose to cause a cancer. Emotional states condition mood and both can influence body function.

The brain is the computer through which all this is modulated and it has various layers and levels of control and response. The probability is that somewhere in the brain a series of reactions take place, based on inheritance, personality and past experience. These will determine the way in which the individual will react to a challenging situation.

Personality-environment equation

We noted right at the beginning that health was difficult to define. WHO got near it by relating health to physical, mental and social well-being. One can go a different way round the course and come up with an answer useful as a working basis for understanding dis-ease. This is what I have called the *personality-environment equation.*

It must by now be inescapable that from, and presumably even before birth, we are all in a state of dynamic reaction with the environment. Each of us perceives the environment differently because of our personalities, etc. Provided that the personality and environment are reasonably in balance there will be no need to opt out and the individual will be healthy. If not, defence reactions will be provoked and he will be dis-eased and uncomfortable.

In terms of business or other life, one can put this slightly differently and say, particularly for the middle aged, that an individual needs to balance his aspirations and his attributes. It is no good driving oneself in a direction or at a speed which one was not designed to go. To do so will be stressful, so will driving too slowly or being underemployed. Ambition must always be tempered by the achievable.

It is true to say that most of the problem areas in the environment come from interpersonal relations and problems made by people and not from physical causes. Unfortunately, people tend to be bad at dealing with each other, particularly in firms and families. Things are said and done for the wrong reasons and there is a tendency to run away from reality and the truth, which in the end causes more difficulty. In our medical work, it is surprising how often people become all steamed up and genuinely ill, without realizing what the fuss is about. Similarly the provoker or initiator of the reaction is frequently quite oblivious of the effect his statement or action is having on the recipient.

Half the battle in dealing with stress is to identify the problem and admit that there is one. Having done this one can set about looking at the options for solving it. The other half of the problem is to have enough insight to know yourself and how you will react, what are your strengths and weaknesses, etc. It is also, especially for people who are responsible for other people, useful to have an awareness as to how your 'signals' are being received down the line. What effect are *you* having on the environment and is it good or bad? Often too, the signal you send out is quite differently received, for right or wrong reasons, which is stressful to others and possibly frustrating for you.

To a degree, frustration is the same as what the psychiatrists call conflict. One gets stuck into a situation, from which there is no obvious way out. Sometimes the conflict is obvious, but often it occurs at a subconscious level. Thus, although it determines perceived behaviour, the chain of cause and effect has been lost. It is often easier to see conflict at work in children. If a child is faced with two alternatives between which he cannot choose or the answers to both are uncongenial, the likelihood is that the child will burst into tears or behave irrationally. Apart from grief, crying or laughter is often the only way of postponing action or relieving tension in a conflicting situation. It is a short-term way to get off the hook; indeed as tension builds up in any situation it has to be released by laughter, tears, a display of violence, or irrational tantrum outburst. One of the difficulties from which managers suffer is that they are expected to appear calm at all times. Their natural responses have to be bottled up or sublimated until they can later go and kick the dog or behave irritably at home.

Fatigue and age

Two final points require to be made in this outline about understanding and living with stress. The first concerns fatigue, which is a separate entity. Tired people are not of necessity stressed, but although it cannot be measured scientifically, there seems to be little doubt that the stress thresholds become lowered by fatigue. Fatigue seems to lower other thresholds like resistance to disease. Also, and this can be serious, it impairs judgement. Thus a tired person will take wrong decisions, or get into difficult situations, or get caught by pitfalls he would normally avoid. The effects of fatigue can thus become extremely stressful.

Age appears to be a factor here. The young are much more resilient and will bounce back more easily. Because of their relative lack of experience of life, they charge ahead without being so aware of the hazards and pitfalls. A corollary of all this is that on the whole the more intelligent a person is, the more likely he is to be stressed. At one or another level of consciousness, the conflict has to be perceived before it becomes potentially harmful. To take an extreme example, the 'soldier' who stops and counts the odds is less likely to be superbrave than the more thick-skinned man who charges regardless into the battle field. Similarly, thick-skinned extroverted people are more likely to cause, and sensitive people more likely to perceive, interpersonal stress. Thus, analytical and critical people are more likely to be stressed than their more extroverted and perhaps less-intelligent *confrères*.

Alternative satisfactions

The second and perhaps more important point concerns the value of alternative sources of satisfaction. Successful people inevitably have high morale, because nothing succeeds like success. Even in the face of great fatigue and anxiety, it is failure or relative failure that causes stress. Thus top people, in spite of the load they carry, tend not to be stressed because they can and are coping.

It is the people below them and those who are not making some of the grade who are likely to be stressed. It is no good judging outstanding people by normal or average standards. On the whole they will only get stressed when things go wrong and then, of course, they fall very hard.

But the trouble with all single-track people is that they remain very vulnerable. As they get older, it is essential for them to acquire alternative interests and satisfactions, so they build up a credit account of high moral to underwrite the work situation.

'Number twos' are frequently more stressed than 'number ones'; they are not in control and get pushed around or do not wholly approve of the way things are done. It is more satisfying to stop the buck than to pass it on. There is more stress in middle than top management. There are two morals to this short tale; the first is the importance of *outside* interests (discussed further in Part Two) and the second is the need to realize the necessity of playing in the right league if one is to avoid stress and this includes too little as well as too much challenge.

A final point about successful tycoons, and for that matter successful other people, is that their work and success is often so demanding that it puts their lives out of balance. They tend to be outstandingly successful in their mainstream activity, but rather poor at some of the other things important in life. For instance, it was found that many of the top people we saw often got more stress and anxiety from their domestic life than they did from their work. They tended to take the former for granted, but really were knocked sideways when, usually predictably, it went sour on them.

This brings me back to the importance of alternative satisfactions. As a rough classification and for purposes of our stress assessment, we divide life into work, home and leisure. Work and home may seem fairly obvious, but why leisure? The answer, particularly from middle age onwards, is simple. The man whose sole interest lies in his work is very vulnerable. With all his eggs in his .work basket he has nothing to fall back on if things at work go wrong. I have laid great emphasis on the fact that the whole of life feeds into the personality-environment equation. Thus, what happens outside work can and must effect what can be put into work, and visa versa. For this and other reasons it is therefore highly desirable that we should all have alternative satisfactions to fall back on. Success in one field will raise morale and help to balance failure in another.

Pleasure obtained from domestic life, the success of children, doing other things well, or being involved in non-work activities, are all essential to balance out life. In addition, of course, the man or woman whose whole life is centred on work is, by middle age, a thundering bore. (For the same reasons, so too is the totally domestically oriented housewife.)

All he can talk about is work and all his contacts and acquaintances relate to his professional life. He really is unnecessarily vulnerable and as part of our effort to improve health, we encourage these people, having looked at themselves metaphorically in the mirror, to develop some outside interests. Some of these should involve exercise in the open air and contact with a different set of people.

By adopting this policy, the man is likely to become rather better at his work because he approaches it more objectively and with better balance. He is healthier, because his equation is in balance too.

Finally, a word of warning: it is tempting, and questions are always being asked round this point, to model oneself on the outstanding people who are brought to one's attention through the professional and other media. But it must be realized that the very great majority of us are ordinary, average people who must, to survive, abide by the ordinary rules. For us to attempt to behave as 'they do' would be disastrous.

In any field the people at the top get there because they have special gifts, attributes and strengths which are not given to a lesser man. Often they get there because they can break the rules and get away with it, but for a variety of reasons it is usually fatal for us to try. We are not in that league.

Stocktaking

Stress can be a special problem in middle age, because if by then one has not learnt to equate personal aspirations with personal attributes, one will be stressed. Equally, if by then one has not learnt to live reasonably sensibly, one is likely to be both stressed and vulnerable.

Two or three years ago, I was addressing a gathering of not very young looking pension-fund managers on stress and related topics. I became very unpopular by suddenly announcing that it might be wise to abandon ambition at 50. This was based on the assumption that most of us, being ordinary, are likely to get stuck on the middle-age ladder; so that round 50 it is sensible to come to terms with what you have got, stop trying quite so hard, and start enjoying other things a bit more. A life that is not on the whole enjoyed is likely to cause dis-ease.

A serious stocktaking is a very good start to life after 50. What have I done so far? What do I want to do with the next 25 years? What are the problem areas? How fit am I (see Chapter 15) and what fences need mending? Unless this is done, or unless you are a very clever chap, you are more likely than not to become increasingly stressed, frustrated and dis-eased, as you get older. Remember happy, well-adjusted people are seldom ill.

Another reason for this stocktaking is that there are several significant watersheds in life; one of them comes in middle age. It is the sudden or gradual awareness of the harsh fact that in many respects you are no longer the resilient, bouncing, go-getting executive of but a few years ago. You still have skills and may take an increased responsibility but you tire more easily and do not bounce back so quickly. There are, you ought to admit, things that younger people do better. You must learn to manipulate the youngsters and not insist on doing it all yourself.

Dealing with stress

The burden of all this is that the key to dealing with stress, particularly as we get older, is firstly to know something of what stress is all about and what the warning signals might mean. The second thing is to try, as honestly as possible, and it is not easy, to know yourself. What are your strengths and weaknesses, how do others see you and what job satisfaction does your wife (should you have one) get out of being married to you?

Another key to dealing with stress is to try to identify the 'stress' or problem. From what *source* does the anxiety and tension, the frustration and the conflict arise. This identification is halfway to solving the problem, it may in fact be unsolvable, like high-interest rates, or the three- or two-day week, but at least it can be pushed to one side to allow one to get on with the rest of life.

Because business is competitive, people at the very top are often very short of 'people' to talk to; this is made worse by the fact that many executives prefer not to talk business to their wives. Maybe too, some wives are incapable of being talked to along these lines. But if one can find some means of exteriorizing and sharing a problem area it immediately makes it better.

But please do not finish up with any idea that I think that this philosophy makes life easy, because I do not and it is not. Life, which consists largely of interpersonal relations and quality judgements, is complicated enough. Running a business in the shifting sands and general political lunacy of today's conditions is hell — only the tough can survive and perhaps only the crazy try. Why, for instance, don't we managers settle for regular hours and more modest salary?

Perhaps it is because some of us want to be stressed, or at any rate put under nearly intolerable strain, to show how clever and tough we are.

SIX

Mental Breakdown

When I was a medical student, our training in psychological medicine consisted of a course of lectures on insanity, visits to a mental asylum (Colney Hatch) and some medico-legal information on the intricacies of certification and how to get hold of a strange but useful gentleman called the Relieving Officer. I went to the lectures and paid one visit to the asylum on a Saturday morning, where there was a standard demo of 'star turns' who ambled amiably on to the platform and solemnly announced that they were the Queen of Sheba, or ate a few razor blades.

Mental disease then was divided roughly into subnormality, due to congenital (born with) brain abnormality, psychotic and neurotic behaviour disorders. The first two required custodial care, probably more for the protection of the rest of the community than for the benefit of the patient. Virtually no treatment, except sedation and straightjackets, was available and there was little understanding of the basic changes which caused the disturbances. Freudian psychoanalysis was practised, but it was very much a minority cult and in any case was conducted by very odd people and seemed to go on forever; looking for 'woodshed type' happenings in early life, to be interpreted in terms of orogenital symbolism.

The term neurotic was applied to those behaviour disturbances, which were obviously nervous, but were not severe enough to require custodial care. Less serious symptoms, for which no organic basis could be found, were called functional, believed not really to exist and, therefore, not conceivably important. The patient was got rid of as expeditiously as possible. Certainly, they were not accepted by doctors as the call for help or manifestation of disease which all symptoms represent.

It is also worth realizing that up to very recently almost half the hospital beds in this country were devoted to mental illness of some sort. The number has only recently been overtly reduced by reducing the designated beds, putting acute mental cases into general wards and discharging patients from institutions and back into the community which is ill equipped to deal with them, thus increasing the stress on both parties.

It was, and to a degree still is, hardly surprising that mental ill health got itself such a bad name that no-one liked to admit suffering from it. Indeed, it is only relatively recently, and the change is still occurring, that people can have a nervous breakdown, depression and so on and survive both socially and medically. But the situation is improving and psychiatrists are becoming both sensible and respectable.

The role of psychiatry

Although there are still tremendous gaps in our knowledge of the functioning of the brain and what goes wrong with it to cause conditions which disrupt personality, like schizophrenia, we do know enough to give us a working knowledge of 'neurotic behaviour'. We also have, which is much more important, a framework, based on classical Freudian and other psychology, as a basis on which we can reasonably successfully treat people psycho-therapeutically. In addition to this, there are also highly successful methods of drug and other treatment such as tranquillizers (which are prescribed, largely unnecessarily, by the ton), sedatives, anti-depressants or other drugs, to say nothing of electric shock therapy and in rare cases brain surgery called leucotomy. The fact is that the chances of treatment now being successful and the almost universal consumption of tranquillizers, have helped to make mental breakdown less unpalatable, ie tranquillizers and psychiatrists can be discussed at cocktail parties.

When I first started clinical work with businessmen, it was still very difficult to persuade someone to go and see a psychiatrist; who had to be misleadingly packaged to become acceptable. This was, of course, largely due to the fact that many of them were very odd birds who said and did rather little and what they did say was either gobble-de-gook or implied that all the patients' problems arose from sex or excretion, or too much or too little of both. An early patient of mine went to a man who described himself as an analytical hypnotist. Being unable to produce the right sort of dreams, my man used to lie on the couch in resentful silence. After several sessions of this, he gave up, complaining bitterly that he was not going to pay ten pounds an hour to be grunted at.

Based on the lines of argument outlined in the last chapter, we do now know a lot more about the reasons for normal and abnormal responses, in terms of the resolution of the personality-environment equation. We also know that drugs and electric shock apart, individuals can be introduced to themselves. Having learnt something of what makes them tick in a certain way, they can be helped either to tick differently or live more tranquilly with something they now understand. This is what psychiatry is concerned with and there is really nothing mysterious about the doctors and fully trained lay people who practice it. Because too, psychiatry now has so much more to offer, it is attracting more credible people, which obviously helps. The days of the head shrinker with a funny accent are passing.

We know that in psychosomatic terms, both behaviour disturbance and overtly painful or disabling symptoms can be explained on the basis of a personality-environment clash producing a basically protective response. One of the things a psychiatrist can do is to discover what one is running away from or why certain situations are uncongenial. Another feature of all this is a greater realization of the importance of conflict and anxiety. The amount of uncertainty, fear and excitement a person can live with is a major feature determining an individual's stability and, to a degree, the style of life that he chooses for himself. Fatigue also lowers the anxiety threshold.

Some causes of breakdown

In order to survive in business, its practitioners must have a very high toleration of anxiety and a willingness to take risks. If they want to play safe, but yet be in industry or commerce, they need to go into a large bureaucratic organization, where they are small cogs within big wheels with little direct responsibility, neither do they have much tangible end product of their work. This is a situation which most of us would find frustrating, but these people tend to settle for the security and say how good the pension is. I used to work for a large and amorphous international oil company, whose London office was packed with relatively senior people, most of whom had failed in overseas jobs. They had high-sounding titles and worked at passing files. Looking back at this, it became apparent that they settled for status and security and got their satisfactions from outside social activity.

Hopefully, it is clear that not only is mental disease part of the whole illness spectrum, but also within the spectrum of mental disease itself, there is a range of behaviour which varies in both abnormality and the amount of disability it produces. Thus, a phobic person who, for instance, cannot bear crowds, can lead a perfectly normal life at home. Someone who cannot fly, can travel by a variety of other routes. These can be very serious disturbances but, provided the limitations they impose are accepted, little disability is caused. Similarly, religious or dietetic bigotry can be limiting to the exent at least of verging on the abnormal as far as behaviour is concerned.

Overt mental breakdown, which disorganizes function is much more dramatic. Thus, someone in an acute anxiety state will develop symptoms like trembling, crying, insomnia, insecurity and inability to do anything coherently. Similarly, the range of depressions already described can be disabling to the point of suicide. Even mild depression interferes with judgement and work capacity.

All these and many more, represent dis-ease, the manifestations of which are emotional or behavioural, rather than physical or painful, but, and to repeat the point, the causes of either set of symptoms are likely to be the same. We also need to remember that individual thresholds vary and that some people are much more stable and less exciteable than others. Some people have no toleration of anxiety and insecurity and fly off the deep end at what seems trivial provocation while others seem to need to generate anxiety about trivial things in order to have something to worry about.

The main ages for moderately severe mental breakdown are adolescence (a period of great emotional instability, learning and discovery), early adult life and late middle age. Thus, one of the hazards of middle age is likely to be the possibility of mild mental breakdown.

From what has been said, this type of dis-ease is likely to occur at times of stress and/or instability. To a degree, this is cumulative and, if middle age has been on the whole disappointing and frustrating, aspirations and attributes not equated, if the appearance of the end of the road is feared, ie retirement, it may precipitate a breakdown; so, of course, may mergers and takeovers.

When we looked at the basic statistics in Chapter 1, one of the minor points was that the commonest cause of death in the younger age group was violence, ie road accidents and suicide. Younger people are more volatile and older people more gloomy. Clinically, one of the most satisfying areas of help is the temporarily over-promoted youngster. Having done reasonably well, perhaps rather too quickly, such a person is suddenly thrown in the deep-end and finds that at least some of the buck stops at him. This may cause loss of confidence from which a whole host of symptoms, which often includes the drinking habit, can ensue. Should this coincide with domestic stress as well, the situation can become potentially destructive, at least as far as the career is concerned.

Thus, and this is the burden of this chapter, if life has gone reasonably well for the individual, middle age should be mentally fairly tranquil. If, on the other hand, the disappointments, the failures and the over-indulgences build up, mental breakdown is a real possibility. A contributory factor here for businessmen is that they are still undertrained professionally (many left school young and made their own way), organizations are overstaffed, there are management consultants, and technical change and takeovers occur. The anxiety and uncertainty produced by all this is obvious and in health terms, can be very unsettling.

Help and rehabilitation

Should the worst occur, it must be realized that individuals who get caught in this trap, can very often be helped and rehabilitated. To achieve this, they themselves, the company and their families must first admit that all is not well and, secondly, seek help. Usually, because of perfectly legitimate pride and lack of insight, the individual involved is reluctant to give up and give in. He has to be prodded in the direction of the salvation by one of the other involved parties. In this respect, it is interesting to note that one of the American leaders of psychosomatic thought ascribes most illness to what he calls the 'given up-giving up syndrome'; helplessness and hopelessness, as it has been called. This does perhaps over-dramatize the situation, but some of his case history descriptions do substantiate the point that much illness is related to giving up.

The earlier action is taken, the greater the chances of success. Mild and severe mental breakdown can now be regarded in exactly the same light as all other comparably debilitating and life-altering disease. Individuals ought to learn from failure and relative failure. I have a patient who is now rapidly becoming the prototype professional chairman. About ten years after the war, he had a mild anxiety breakdown, due largely to overwork. This was, for him, a very salutary experience and he is totally determined that it will never happen again.

Decline in confidence

An interesting area of speculation as regards middle-aged behaviour concerns virility and general performance, in relation to age. Why is it that, on the one hand, there are a few people who go on well after the age of 70 in full control of their faculties and with judgement and enthusiasm unimpaired? Such people are nearly always outstanding and at the top of their respective trees. On the other hand, one also meets, probably more frequently, the man who did immensely well up to middle age. He was an articulate, lively go-getter, of whom great things were expected, but suddenly he is transformed into a rather bumbling prevaricative administrator who has to be pushed into the simplest decisions.

The first man was built differently, seems determined to go on forever and looks like being able so to do. There is some evidence that one of the factors contributing to this is a continuing high male hormone output. However, do not get too hopeful as there is no hard evidence that hormone boosts will reverse the trend in you!

What suddenly turns the men in the second group sour is not known. It must be some mental or hormonal change which has destroyed their confidence. Two others factors certainly contribute. The first is that the man was probably over-promoted and over-rated in his early assessment, ie he was not really a high flyer. The second is that he may have got burnt out too soon. A contributory factor could also be the male menopause, which is not fully understood but does occur.

Late middle age, particularly, is the period of pay-off. If life has been reasonably successful and not too demanding, retirement will be approached with tranquillity. If, on the other hand, the individual has been struggling against the tide, the pay-off will come. If he does not get a coronary or some other organic disease, a 'nervous breakdown' may ensue. What then is a nervous breakdown? It is a defence situation in which for any one of a variety of reasons the individual ceases to be able to function coherently. It is all rather shaming; he may tremble, cry, laugh hysterically or just sit. In minor forms decision taking and general effectiveness suffer. Alternatively, there may be a drift into depression or alcoholism, because of disillusionment and disappointment with life and an inability to face the future.

Mental breakdown which can take a variety of forms but it is worth remembering that plenty of people have survived worse crises and that with understanding and modern therapeutic methods the outlook is usually good.

PART TWO
SURVIVING THE HAZARDS

SEVEN
Dealing with Executive Stress

The message of this book is to make the point that for most people reasonable health is mainly dependent on two factors. Firstly, living sensibly and not too indulgently and secondly, enjoying what you do and how you live. Part Two is about the second area. This can be summarized by repeating the underlying assertion that happy, well-adjusted people are seldom ill.

We have seen that although 'life is for living', it must also be challenging in one of a variety of ways and at several levels. A very thoughtful and successful post-war manager started his working life on the shop floor doing extremely boring and repetitive work. He used to keep reasonably motivated and sane by setting himself production targets by the half day. Thus, if he was feeling a bit off colour, he set a lower target. Presumably, all this was before the days when the unions decreed how hard an individual should work and how much he was allowed to earn.

The other point he used to make, which has always stuck in my mind, was his statement that if everyone then working for him did not know what the company was about, and what it was doing, he had failed as a manager. In these days of philosophizing about business and management, this may sound a crashing platitude but, in fact, how many executives do know where they are going, how they fit in and what the future might hold? This is one of the things that reasonable adjustment is all about.

It is much easier for the outsider, be he industrial journalist, management consultant or doctor, to take the pulse of an organization. Those who live with and in it, particularly if they have been there for some years, get so used to the climate that they tend not to notice it. Yet it is true to say that no two organizations, even if they are part of a unified group, are identical. Each has its own specific climate and traditions, the climate being largely determined by the interplay between the personalities, or personality, of the people at the top and the traditions of the organization.

Successful job matching

Given that the individual has at some time a range of choice, and he is seldom so desperate that he has to take any job, it behoves him or his advisers, and, if they have the sense, those who appoint him, to try to ascertain whether his personality will fit into the existing climate. If it does not, there may well be considerable stress and the 'marriage' is less likely to work out. Thus a successful job match depends firstly on the candidate having the requisite skills and, secondly, fitting reasonably well into the interpersonal climate.

One tough buccaneering firm in high technological manufacturing needed well-qualified technologists and tended to recruit rather pale, genteel, university graduates. At their pre-employment medicals they were always in impeccable order medically, but, after a couple of years in the environment into which they were going, they became disillusioned wrecks. Having seen something of what happened to them, later, as I took them out into the street, I used to say, 'Please don't quote me on this, but my personal advice to you is not to go and work for that outfit. Tempting though the job is, you are not the right sort of animal for that jungle. They are likely to chew you up and spew you out'. Swashbuckling extroverts, however, did splendidly.

Tyzack once told me about a very painful time he had with a smallish family company, looking for a new and bright managing director. They were all competent self-made men and they thought that what they needed was a more gentlemanly university graduate. Basically an excellent idea, but how would he, as the only one of his species, fit in with them? Tyzack convinced them that it might be better for both if he looked for someone who had come up the hard way.

Business life is full of anecdotes and folklore about idiosyncratic characters who made good and also made a lot of money. They were usually the outstanding people who got away with breaking all the rules. Much less is heard about the often very hard life that was led by those who had to work close to them. Although the financial rewards were usually high, they had to be to attract people, it was often a dog's life with a high morbidity rate.

Dominant managers

There is also a more insidious form of domination which is in no way harsh or combative, but tends to drive out the really good people who are not tolerated as equals. Indeed sitting on the sidelines, particularly after a merger, one can predict that once the honeymoon is over a new pecking order will be established and that a number of people will be looking for alternative jobs. This sort of situation is, of course, grist for the headhunters.

In this sort of behaviour pattern, there used to be a very few tycoons who apparently took a malicious pleasure in seemingly setting out to destroy people by undermining their self-confidence. Theoretically, it was always possible to stand up to the boss, but this produced such flaming rows and, after all, he was the boss running the shop his way.

It is very much part of the capitalist ethic that individuals can create organizations in their own image and that other individuals can take or leave the climate as they choose. As business life is so much more complicated than it used to be, it tends to need more technically competent people. As this type of person tends to have a choice, the behaviour of the firm has to be at least partially modified to attract people, so that this is a situation which is probably less common than it was.

Reference has been made already to the influence that lack of insight into the effect of a senior person's behaviour and decisions can have on those for whom he is responsible. Many people are unaware of what they do to others and a lot of organizations are less happy and probably less effective because of the upset and tension that this produces. To give a very simple and rather pathetic example, we were doing an executive health scheme for a small firm of about six rather unhappy people. We were asked also to see the chairman's personal assistant, a rather sad middle-aged women with recurrent abdominal pain, which had so far defied the usual diagnostic investigations. When we got her talking, it was apparent that she was terrified of going to the lavatory because whenever she was absent for more than a few minutes at a time, her boss put his finger on the buzzer. She was merely, but severely, constipated.

I went with the doctor concerned to see the chairman to talk to him about this and other discontents which were unsettling the group. He was superficially at least, overcome with remorse, said he would mend his ways, and soon expunged his guilt with a pay rise.

In human terms, the trouble with this type of situation is that it is the meek, second-rate or averagely average people who tend, because of age and lack of formal qualification, to get stuck unhappily into these uncongenial climates. Mostly all that can be done is to encourage them to develop alternative satisfactions in activities outside their work. Obviously, it is very much easier to preach or comment about these situations than it is to alter or improve them, but the issue has been raised because it has two important implications. The first, and we shall come back to it, is that anyone who is responsible for other people ought to look over his shoulder and try to assess what they, as well as he, stand to gain. The development of more professional management over the past ten years has, in fact, improved this situation.

The second and perhaps more useful point is that everyone must realize that there are 'horses for courses'. In any employment or promotion situation, the question of interpersonal as well as technical fit should be asked. Should a mistake have been made, it is, on the whole, worth a lot of trouble to try to alter it with goodwill and without loss of 'face'. But this type of situation, the wrong man in the interpersonal situation, can and does cause an immense amount of preventable stress. (Often it is no-one's fault; it was how they were made).

Sometimes it is said of certain top business people that if they gave half as much attention to interpersonal relations and communication as they did to making money, they might make even more money. They might also with benefit pay more attention to their families. It is difficult to understand how this type of person survives without, if not being clouted, at least being stood up to and told off. A lot of stress would be saved if the stiff upper lip was encouraged to curl a little and allowed to utter a few home truths. Climates could be enormously improved by providing an opportunity for people to say what they think about each other rather than harbour grievances. The long-harboured grievance has a habit of becoming a chip on the shoulder and becoming very stressful. I am a great protagonist, and it gets me into continual trouble, of more plain speaking. This also has the advantage of unclouding some of the options.

Another way in which horses get on to the wrong course is by promotion into a different stream. Many young men join industry as professionally qualified technicians. They do well and having got to the top of their particular bit of the ladder, the next promotional step is away from their expertise into more general management. This inevitably involves people rather than things or ideas. Very often they have no training for this and the results can be disastrous, both for the individual and those under him.

It is an underrated fact that the success of most organizations depends on someone's ability to motivate people and get them to identify with the organization. Like a marriage, there has to be enough in the relationship for both parties to make it worthwhile and productive. Even in the best run company, there is more than enough challenge for everyone without frittering away precious energy on stressful friction and frustration.

Role Ambiguity

Another major form of institutional stress is what the social scientists call role ambiguity. It is astonishing, particularly in quite large organizations, how many people do not really know what they are meant to be doing and what their responsibilities actually are. This is also true at the very top of organizations of all sizes. Full-time executive directors, for instance, often get their policy-making directorial roles hopelessly mixed up with their executive managerial role. Not only does this produce administrative confusion, but it is also quite clear to any perceptive observer that there is no real policy. The so-called board lurches about from one *ad hoc* decision to another. Situations like this, which are not uncommon, can cause a great deal of stress, particularly at middle management level. No clear message ever emerges from the confusion upstairs.

Another cause of confusion is the misuse of the appointment or post of 'director'; directorships get distributed with gay abandon to keep people happy. One particular large company grew by taking over smaller concerns all over the country. The previous owners, of quite small businesses, were given good money and made directors of the new and much larger company. It soon became a fleet staffed almost exclusively with admirals. One day I saw a very frustrated and moderately senior member of this outfit who complained bitterly that he could not even get equipment for his staff. When I said, 'Look you are a director of the company and you can authorize this expenditure, do it without telling anyone, and see what happens', he was horrified, but it worked. The other thing this company did was to make the senior salesmen 'directors', because they thought that this impressed the customers. Perhaps it did if the customers were stupid enough but it caused great role ambiguity in the individuals.

Not everyone in industry and commerce either wants, or is equipped, to be a general. Many people want a reasonably rewarding life and to know what they are expected to do and be able to get on and do it. In every organization there ought to be someone whose job it is to make sure that the staff at all levels have both a job description and something definably productive to do. Two other items need to be included in this overview. The first is to be on the look out for areas of interpersonal friction and tension and the other is to try to adjust the challenge locally to the needs and the abilities of those concerned. As we have seen, over promotion can cause stress because the individual cannot inherently cope; if he cannot cope, of course, things also go wrong because of the interpersonal or administrative constraints in the system. However, for a bright person to be underemployed is almost the most stressful thing that can happen. It is extremely frustrating and disaffecting.

Tyzack and I used to separate executives into two main groups which we called small- and large-firm men. The former tended to be much more entrepreneurial and, to a degree, was happy to be a big fish in a small pond. He needed excitement, identity and close contact with the sharp end. He expected the rewards to be high, but had a limited interest in pensions and security.

The large-firm man tended to be a bureaucrat and, on the whole, happy to be a smaller fish in a much larger pond and to be dominated by the system which he had no interest in changing. Obviously, there are variants of these two basic types, but if the wrong man strays into the wrong slot, which he may well do in answering an advertisement to a tempting looking job, it is stressful for the individual and the organization.

A somewhat similar situation occurs when the needs of a company change. One man may be good at creating and building up an activity. It then needs consolidating by another type of person. After ten years or so, consolidators tend to get stuck and perhaps become a bit complacent; they need digging out and replacing by a go-getter or rebuilder. The need for all these types of change and the effects of not dealing with them, or handling the situation badly, can again be stressful.

Source of Power

In any organization or situation, power resides at certain focal points or in the hands of usually one individual. There is nearly always a difference between the way power is exercised *de facto* and *de jure*. When it comes to the crunch, things may appear to happen, quite predictably for seemingly the wrong reasons. Before starting on a situation or embarking on a piece of intrigue, it is wise to do some homework and to make a ruthlessly realistic assessment of where power or decision taking really resides. Obvious answers to management situations are few and far between; usually there are several possible courses of action and it is necessary that ultimately attitudes should be polarized and sides taken. If, however, it is a situation in which one is vitally concerned or about which has strong views, it is foolish to push these too far in the face of reality. Defeat or frustration is stressful.

Frustration and lack of confidence in the man above you are sadly common and there is an inevitable tendency to go round or over him. Rows may be provoked and a lot of geat generated, but the people who do this get very hurt when, in the ultimate, the system backs the hierarchy. A dim or dead-beat senior will nearly always defeat a bright and frustrated junior. It is astonishing how often individuals come unstuck because they somehow think that when it comes to them, the rules of power do not matter — they do. Virtue is hierarchical.

In most human activities, there is a need for competition and a hierarchical arrangement of power and responsibility. Competition is not only between organizations but, inevitably, it is also between individuals within the organization. Provided this is kept reasonably civilized, it is productive and, in any case, there is no alternative to it. Leaderless groups and collective responsibility may produce highly identified participants, but they tend to waste time and make little progress. Talking becomes an end in itself.

In planning and running an organization a balance has to be held between competitive challenge and too much kindly security. It is good but not essential to have everyone happy; some insecurity tends to make people try and work harder. On the other hand, too much ruthless disregard of the needs and requirements of others can destroy people and in the end the ruthless will have to be replaced.

Delegation

One of the problems of growing old gracefully, particularly if fairly senior, is that of delegation. Like the technocrat turning manager, the line manager, particularly if he has come up the hard way, tends to be a doer. He likes to get stuck into situations and 'get his hands dirty'. When he gets promoted to policy-making management — a role he does not really understand — he wants to charge about doing things and will not give anyone a chance to get on by themselves. It is worth remembering that one cannot do as much as one gets older. A favourite question when investigating this situation is to ask the man concerned what he thinks it would be like 'working for him' in those conditions. To reduce stress on oneself and provide satisfaction for others, there must be jobs down the line which are satisfying for good people to do.

Delegation is easy to preach but hard to achieve in practice, but it is essential from our point of view. On the whole only secure people can delegate power and responsibility. Insecure people, who subconsciously do not dare to give anything away, are impossible to work for. They are stressed because they are overworked and worried about their status, etc, and their associates are stressed because they are mucked about and obviously not trusted to do anything that matters.

In all this interpersonnel interplay, confrontation, even if it is abrasive and outspoken, is more productive than the hypocrisy of the half truth and the evasive answer. Good vigorous discussion, even if it generates heat, can be a valuable asset. People have got to learn to disagree and even be defeated without bearing grudges. But the decision having been taken, must be seen to be implemented and not quietly sabotaged from above. If this occurs, everyone will stop trying.

Frustration

A last cause of environmental stress is boredom. Middle managers particularly tend to get stuck in a rut. They know their jobs backwards, and it is mutually convenient for both parties to leave them there until they retire. One firm had an infinitely worthy and competent cost and works accountant who had about ten more years to work with the firm and could not conceivably be promoted. However, he turned up a year or so later looking a changed, brighter and more cheerful man. He had been moved sideways into a different department and made to learn a new job.

People need change and new challenge and individuals and organizations would benefit enormously from more 'sideways promotion'. Similarly, the men who spend all or most of their life in one organization are very vulnerable. After many years they are unsaleable to anyone else and even if quite senior tend to be well glued to the bottom of the company rut. The impression is that to remain young and lively, no-one, particularly as they get older, should be allowed to go on doing the same job for more than ten years. He becomes a menace to himself and the organization. A change of job every decade should be the motto.

A new hazard, or at least a different climate to which a good deal of adaptation may be required, is the multi-national organization, and not far removed from this is the conglomerate. It seems fair to link them together because they both share the same weakness, namely the distance between the top of the pyramid, where decisions are taken and capital allocated, and the bottom of the heap, where some poor and still hopefully entrepreneurial executive is out on a limb trying to get things done with no authority to buy a bottle of ink without asking someone in America. A bemused doctor trying to entice a secretary into the London medical department of a vast American oil company rang me one day. He was being told by New York the salary he could pay and that she was not to have more than two weeks holiday, neither of which decisions had any relation to the local market rate.

American companies are, or until recently used to be, very bad about this type of behaviour. Their dedication to systems and philosophies produced layers of middle management, made up of 'no men' who created nothing and existed to stop other people doing anything. Large organizations are inevitably bureaucratic and international ones particularly so. Very few companies seem to have solved the problem of size in relation to delegation and controls. The job may glitter on paper, but it is a demanding climate to live in and it does require a certain type of animal, possibly someone who has been through a business school and learnt the jargon and part of the philosophy.

A good friend of mine took over as managing director of an American engineering company in this country. It was also a family dominated group. Two days after taking office he received long and detailed cables about what they expected him to do. He replied quite tersely, inquiring who was running the UK subsidiary. If they wanted to do it, it was a waste of his time and their money for him to sit and answer cables. He was a strong enough person to take a tough line, and he was also outstandingly able, but I have seen several people almost destroyed by petty bullying from America. Being rung up through the night, and pursued round Europe with trivial messages, does not make for equanimity. One man was disturbed three times in a morning while trying to conduct some extremely complicated labour negotiations in Rome. In his judgement the queries were totally unnecessary and could have been put on his desk in London.

The only way to control this situation is to be tough, difficult, and dictate your own terms. To succeed at this, requires great ability otherwise you are doomed. If you cannot win, it is probably better to get out before you blow a gasket. Running any company under today's conditions is difficult enough, but to be behoven to a bureaucracy in another country, who have seemingly no understanding of local problems and conditions, can be tantamount to murder, and it is also a very insecure life. The money may seem good, but life expectancy is often limited. A great deal of dis-ease arises from entanglements of this kind.

Much of what has been said in this section may appear obvious to the perceptive reader, but he can be assured that the type of situation referred to occurs frequently enough 'in life' to bring it to clinical attention as a significant cause of stress in the business environment.

In this chapter, even if it is adumbrating the obvious, I hope to have developed a little more insight into, and understanding of, the environmental pressures and pitfalls in business life. Given this better understanding it is hoped that individuals will be able to avoid some of them, and that the knowledge of 'what goes' and what they need will help them to drive a better bargain with their working environment. In addition it is hoped that some of the down-trodden 'stressed' will become a bit more militant. One of the best ways of dramatically altering the climate is to say one of the things that everyone thinks, but no-one dares to mention.

EIGHT

Travel

Some years ago I saw a man who was the sales manager of a medium-sized firm, he drove about 50 000 miles a year including regular trips to Scotland up the A1 before it was improved. He told the usual story about this being a comfortable and convenient way to get about and collect his thoughts. In fact, he was running away from life, which could not catch up with his relative failure when he was on the road. The man was rather shocked when I pointed out to him, and later to his managing director, that it was a waste of his not-inconsiderable salary to spend it on sitting behind the steering wheel of a motor car.

Last year, the chief executive of a very large organization, aged 62, who was not an experienced globe trotter, arrived in the consulting room in a state of exhaustion. A month before he had set out for New Zealand to decide whether or not to close down a factory. He went via the West Coast of America and stopped off in Vancouver. Here, he arrived in the early afternoon local time, which was not far off his natural bedtime. While his wife put her feet up, he was whisked off to a business meeting followed by a cocktail party and dinner. Later he was poured onto the night 'plane going west at about the time he should have been having breakfast. It took him a week to recover when he got to Auckland and, at his age and seniority, not only ought he to have known better but also to have set a better example for his younger colleagues.

Travel is now so simple that it tends to be taken for granted, but even considerable transit within this country imposes strain and causes extra fatigue. I feel very strongly that the conditions under which all staff travel, from junior salesmen in Morris 1100s, to the chairman going to New York, should be periodically considered by management and suitable rules laid down.

For those whose work inevitably involves a great deal of travel, which takes them away from home and gets them back worn out, travel becomes a way of life. It also becomes a factor which limits life, or what is left of it after fifty, and thus must be controlled.

Because this is an important but neglected facet of business or company life, it is worth looking at the problems in some detail. It is convenient to do this under the following main headings:

1 Travel within the UK
2 European and short distance travel
3 Worldwide travel against time
4 Effect of travel on the family

But, first, let us look in a little more detail at the nature of travel and what it might do to people. Much of this argument may sound so simple as to be platitudinous, but it is surprising how seldom the implications of travel are properly thought through.

The average man lives at home, goes to work and gets back in the evening. He operates in a familiar environment and to a regular routine. To break this for a day or two is often exciting and stimulating and not bad for the family either, but once the absences become regular, say several days, a fortnight, weeks, a month, or even only home for weekends, a different life pattern is imposed.

This new pattern involves the strain of travel, be this by road, rail or air; the bore of living in hotels with only food, drink and possibly women for relaxation; absence from home; possibly time change and much greater strain of selling, negotiating, representing, etc; away from familiar surroundings; often feeling tired, lost and lonely. To do this regularly, imposes considerable strain on a man and his family and it is important to see that the short-term load does not reduce the long-term expectation of life. A well-run company has an obligation to see that it does not burn out its executives prematurely.

Anyone who has waited at Rome Airport in a strike or at London Airport in a fog, indeed at London or New York Airports under any circumstances, knows that this is a strain much greater than getting to the office at 9.30 a.m.

Quite fortuitously, I met a social anthropologist standing in a queue on a Sunday morning at Rome Airport. We were both hoping to catch a connection to Nice to attend the same conference. There was a strike on and neither of us could understand a word the loudspeaker said. 'There is nothing' he observed dryly, 'like an absent aeroplane to make a business tycoon, bereft of his chauffeur and secretary, feel lost, angry and naked,' I found it frustrating and exhausting as well.

In the United Kingdom

Commercial travellers, notwithstanding all the fancy titles they are now given, are paid to be on the road. If they did not on the whole enjoy it, they would not do the job. The good and ambitious ones get on and up fairly rapidly, the average ones present two sets of problems, neither of which are really related to travel. The first is what to do with them as they get older, as selling methods and philosophies change to their resentment and confusion. The second is that many of them hate being promoted into the area sales office.

The main problem of travel within this country, particularly for the more senior people with whom we are predominantly concerned in this book, is to make sure that travel is by the most appropriate route. It is only very recently that the middle management traveller has learnt to abandon his car and the more senior man to demand, if necessary, a chauffeur. Several years ago we used to see large numbers of people who drove themselves 30-50 000 miles a year. If you work this out, it adds up to a great deal of time on the road. We still ask all the people we see what their annual mileage is, because like commuting, it can be a waste of life. If a man is being paid over £6 000 a year, to spend most of his time in transit, it behoves someone to make sure that the money is well spent and that this much travel is really necessary for this man.

At the Institute of Directors, one of the first exercises we got involved in years ago, was to do with a rapidly expanding and decentralized company. All the directors seemed to be in orbit most of the time, dealing with problems at the factories or distributing centres. One could not escape the conclusion that this had become a way of life and that there was a large element of escape from reality in their behaviour pattern. They looked for fires to rush off and extinguish.

But it is essential to make sure that individuals on the whole go by train or 'plane rather than car and are met and looked after on arrival. Anyone who is paid more than about £10 000 and who really has to drive more than, say, 15 000 miles a year, even from home to work, merits a chauffeur. Driving in and out of London and other large centres, is tiring and frustrating and, although drivers do tell themselves that driving is conducive to thought, sitting in the back dealing with papers, reading the paper or even dozing is a better use of valuable time and energy.

My sociological colleague, Jack Winkler, recently obtained some interesting figures about the effect of executive travel on work schedules. From these there was no doubt that even relatively simple 'within the country' travel lengthened the day appreciably. Not only is there an inevitable tendency to leave earlier and get home late, there is also the problem of coping with the ordinary work which would have otherwise been done. Getting out and about is sensible and desirable, but it must be ensured that it does not impose too much of a burden. And its effect on family life must also be borne in mind.

Within Europe

Travel within Europe, usually by air, by flights of mostly up to three hours and often much shorter duration, presents quite different problems to longer flights eastwards and westwards. European travel is mostly north or south and involves minimum time shift. This means that the day is not seriously distorted and that there is only the normal fatigue and anxiety of travel to deal with.

It tends to be forgotten that for many people and their families, constant air travel is a source of anxiety. One of the most typical cases of psychosomatic stress disease was a lady with severe allergic dermatitis of her hands. She saw numerous doctors and was tested for sensitivity to all the usual detergents and household chemicals. Wearing rubber gloves did not help.

At last her perceptive doctor noticed that the rash always broke out when her husband went away. The doctor told her to come and see him immediately the husband next left. He was surprised to discover that the rash actually started on her ring finger under her wedding ring. This woman had considerable anxiety about being left alone and possibly becoming a widow through an air crash. But in order not to bother her already harassed husband, she never shared her anxiety with him.

Although not inherently difficult, the actual process of short-haul air travel is nothing like as comfortable and convenient as the airlines would have one think. Airports are inconveniently situated, parking is often impossible, 'planes are late, overcrowding in lounges is serious, information hard to come by and telephones difficult to operate. All this, plus the natural anxiety of travel, the stress of dealing with foreigners and living in hotels, etc, places considerable extra strain on the individual. A day or a week spent away, or in travel, must be more tiring than the average day or week at the office. Negotiations are best conducted in English through an interpreter, unless the manager is fluent in the language.

Travellers should stay at central hotels, be encouraged to use taxis or hired cars, 'phone up home regularly and, above all, be back by Friday. With travelling in Europe becoming more prevalent, there is a growing tendency for the executive's weekend to be eroded away.

Management should insist that these people are home by Friday night and do not leave again until Monday morning. They should be met at the airport and driven home in the company car. This is much less tiring than getting to the terminal and then home from there. If the job involves a lot of travel, the man should be assisted to move to an area near the airport. Most organizations try reasonably hard to help their staff and save money by using tourist class travel for journeys of up to four hours or within Europe. This is sensible, but the regular traveller should be allowed the occasional luxury of a first class seat at the end of a long week.

People who travel tend to be over-conscientious and work harder than they would at home. To some extent, they need to be protected from themselves by sensible travel rules laid down by management and made part of the organization's traditional behaviour pattern — what is desirable for European travel is essential for longer journeys.

Against time

No sensible company or individual would expect to take major decisions at 3 o'clock in the morning after a long and gruelling day. Yet politicians in our House of Commons attempt this consistently and travellers leap off aeroplanes and, because the sun is shining, go enthusiastically, if bemusedly, straight into difficult negotiations.

One of the more idiosyncratic and powerful American tycoons, chairman of a vast international conglomerate, is alleged, when visiting Europe, to keep his watch on East Coast time and make his acolytes fit in with him. This strikes me as being, if only from his point of view, a sensible use of power. Recent research has shown that there is a measurable and considerable deterioration in intellectual performance following shift of time base.

It has been said that the US Government has forbidden its officials to go straight off 'planes into meetings. President Nixon certainly set a good example by having two night stops on his way to Peking. Modern communications technology and the pressure and status symbolism of being seen to be living with it, can impose very considerable and undesirable strain on the traveller who is caught up in the rat race. Sensible companies lay down firm rules to protect themselves from poor decisions and their staff from overstrain. Dr Kissinger is clearly the exception that proves the rule.

The problem of long distance travel can be looked at under the following headings and because it is so important and so often neglected, the situation and the limitations on behaviour that it imposes, are worth discussing in some detail.

1 Biological limitations
2 Travel schedules and the outward journey
3 Behaviour while away
4 The return journey
5 Effect on the family (to be discussed in the last section).

Biological limitations: circadian rhythm

Have you ever paused to think why your body works so smoothly and how it is that you wake up, go to sleep, feel hungry, excrete and so on, at regular and predetermined intervals? One's biological *status quo* and basic behaviour pattern is determined by a series of conditioned reflexes and finely adjusted hormone responses. Thus, the body runs down at the end of the day, the supply of various stimulant hormones is reduced, body temperature drops and various other changes associated with sleep and re-charging the batteries take place.

All this is controlled on the basis of an in-built 24-hour biological clock and is called the body's circadian rhythm. It gives all the various systems an in-built time base. If then one suddenly flies to the West Coast of America with a time change of plus eight hours on a 14-15 hour flight, the natural rhythm is turned more or less inside out. Day is turned into night and the body is asked to eat when it should be asleep, be intelligent when it is used to relaxing and so on.

Detailed biochemical and other research has shown that the body takes at least five days to reset its clock after a major shift in time base. Until this has occurred, there is a deterioration in performance and limitation of well-being. To do nothing for five days after arrival is asking too much of most busy people. An appreciable amount of acclimatization however, does occur in 24-36 hours, so that if sensible travel rules are observed, a fair compromise can be made.

In the old days of crossing the Atlantic by boat or the USA by train, the day lengthened or shortened by an hour or two. Major time changes occur on east/west flights (days become longer) and west/east flights (days become shorter). Some people say that going east is more demanding, but there is no firm evidence for this. I suspect that from England going east is mostly 'coming home' and the end of a trip is always more tiring than the beginning.

Flying roughly north and south imposes little time change and depending on Summer Time, etc, London to Johannesburg or Cape Town causes little biological upset, although it is as far away as America.

There is, in addition, the need to make allowances for the more usual changes of climate, culture, currency, language and so on. Soon after the war, before these problems were properly understood, I worked for an oil company in a not very hot but humid area near the equator. Elderly directors and VIP visitors escaping the English winter, inappropriately clad in thick suits, used to be close to collapse at the welcome cocktail party. Travellers must plan their schedules to allow a minimum period of acclimatization.

Outward schedules

A friend and colleague, who is a regular annual visitor to Australia, had recently to make an emergency trip to Sydney to decide whether or not to risk a large sum of money in a property venture. Being experienced and, to some extent, a disciple, he scheduled a 15-day trip to be 5 days in Sydney. He did this for two reasons: first, because he needed to be 'on form' for the negotiations, second, because although this was an emergency, he still saw this fortnight as part of a tough year's programme and he knew that it would be stupid to upset the rest of his year's work by getting seriously over-tired before his next holiday was due.

On a trip to the West Coast of America last year, I arranged to arrive at 8 pm local time, sleep for 12 hours and spend the next day sightseeing sleeping and gently preparing the lecture I had gone there to give.

Travel schedules are too important to be left to travel agents; they should always be checked by an experienced senior staff member to make sure that the rules are being observed. For instance, in the 'Australia trip schedule' on p. 108, it will be seen that the return flights were appreciably longer than the outward ones.

One man's schedule

The managing director of a medium-sized company recently went to Australia at very short notice to make major decisions about a new project running into several million pounds. He normally made an annual, but more leisurely trip, so he was well aware of the difficulties and pitfalls. Figure 8:1 shows his schedule:

		Time change	Journey time
Day 1	Dep London 14.20	+7	15 h 45 min
Day 2	Arr Bangkok 13.05		
Day 3	Free in Bangkok		
Day 4	Dep Bangkok 08.00	+4	10 h 25 min
	Arr Sydney 22.45		
Day 5	Relatively free in Sydney		
Days 6, 7, 8, 9	Very tough negotiating in Sydney		
Day 10	Dep Sydney 13.45		
	Arr Bangkok 21.30	−4	
Day 11	Free in Bangkok		
	Dep 23.20		
Day 12	Arr Amsterdam 10.50	−6	17 h 30 min
Day 13	Amsterdam with wife		
Day 14	Dep Amsterdam 12.00	−1	55 min
	Arr London 11.55		
Day 15	Catching up on papers at home		
Day 16	Back in the office		

Figure 8:1 Schedule for business trip to Australia

This is roughly 14 days away for 5 days work in Sydney. It may appear to some to be an extravagant expenditure of time, but seen in relation to a tough year's work and the need for middle-aged senior managers not to get overtired and irritable, it represents a sensible schedule.

Day 1 was unnecessary and represented a wrong choice of flights. The first rule is that no one stage should involve more than a 7-8 hour time change, this usually implies a 15-16 hour flight. Eight to ten hours flying should be regarded as a normal day's work. There should then be a 24-36 hour stop at a not too uncongenial place, to allow the first stage of acclimatization to take place. The schedule reproduced on my colleague's trip to Sydney illustrates this well. He flew to Bangkok where he had two nights and roughly 36 hours doing nothing. He then flew on to Sydney where he had a further day and two more nights to collect his thoughts before getting seriously involved in negotiations. Coming back, he did much the same thing, except that his wife met him in Amsterdam for a short sight-seeing trip and catching up session.

Flight schedules should be chosen so as to arrive at the end of the day local time. For instance, it seems convenient to get into New York, or anywhere else for that matter, between 6.30 and 9.00 pm local time. This is round midnight biological time. A practice which I strongly recommend is to take a stiff drink, a good strong slug of sleeping pill and reckon not to surface until 7 or 8 the next 'local time' morning. This gives a good start towards recovery. Without artificial aids, there is a dreary tendency to wake between 4 and 5 am and wonder what to do.

It is, however, far too easy to leave London so as to arrive in New York in the early evening or late afternoon whereupon one is met and sucked into local social or business activity. An early bed, even by their standards, still means a very late night by one's own time base and the consequent need to try to eat and digest in the middle of the night.

A good rule is to insist on at least one good night before work on the East Coast of America; two nights and a day off for the West Coast, ie 4 and 7-8 hours time change respectively; and two pauses of at least 36 hours and two nights each for Australia or further. The same should be done coming back. This may sound extravagant, but in fact it represents a prudent husbanding of resources, particularly for regular travellers.

Long journeys should be done, if possible by first-class travel, although if there is space, three tourist seats give more sleeping room than two first. First class, however, does give more room to work, move around, get drinks, choose food, wash and shave, etc. It also tends to represent less bustle and anxiety at airports. One experienced traveller, who did several expensive trips to Australia and Japan per year, carried a credit card and was prepared to transfer forwards whenever the tourist class was too crowded.

My top score in ludicrous class distinction was the pompous chairman, travelling to Australia with his sales director, who insisted that the latter went tourist while 'himself' went up front. The man who had to do the work arrived by far the most exhausted!

On the flight, wear light comfortable clothes, which do not worry too much about business respectability and bear a working relationship to the temperature on arrival. Slippers are a help and so are the eye shades provided for sleep. (Travelling first class recently, I was successful in getting a vote in favour of switching off the taped music that was driving most of us crazy during a prolonged 'in plane', on the ground delay.)

Eating and drinking on long flights should be circumspect. Do not drink more than you would on a normal rather relaxed day at home. Eat one lightish meal as near your normal lunch or dinner time as possible and eschew anything more than a snack at the end of the flight. One's digestion acclimatizes better when empty. Planes tend to be dehydrating and an increased (bland) fluid intake, for example orange juice, is desirable.

Remember that although pressurized, etc, there is less oxygen in the aeroplane's environment than at ground level. A mixture of barbiturate sleeping pill, some tranquillizers and alcohol can considerably lower the body's capacity to use oxygen. This can be dangerous for the weak hearted or hypertensive and airlines quietly but regularly bury a number of passengers who die from this cause every year. It is a safe rule not to take more than one drink with any sort of pill. But on long flights, pills do help sleep and relaxation and regular travellers are well advised to find the dose that suits them.

Some people sleep better than others on 'planes, but inevitably it is low grade and inadquate sleep. Any deficiency has to be made up for on arrival.

It is usually false econonomy not to go by taxi from the airport and certainly a good central hotel is desirable. As already mentioned, at least one night's sound sleep is essential before any serious activity. Unless you are a good natural sleeper, it is wise to take sleeping pills, for example two for the first two nights and one the third. This regime helps to get you acclimatized to the local time sleep rhythm.

While away

Most travellers are both conscientious and want to get home as soon as possible. (Friends and families may think that going to Australia is like going on holiday, but the professional traveller knows better.) Thus there is a tendency to work longer hours and harder than when at home. This may be acceptable on short trips, but for anything longer than a week, steps should be taken to limit hours of work. Entertaining and being entertained counts very much as work.

Those who travel regularly will confirm that discipline over diet, sleep, exercise and so on, plays a handsome dividend. Particularly, until fully acclimatized, insist on being in bed by 11 pm. I found that on a long trip, hostesses and others appreciate this, particularly if they are warned in advance. It is often useful to play off social and personal engagements against business ones, and *vice versa*, so as to get a free evening.

Start the day late; you will be much more popular if the man you are going to see has had time to deal with his post. Walk to his office if this is practicable and insist on 20 minutes exercise a day. Avoid staying in people's houses, except at weekends, and try to get an hour with your feet up before an evening date. This is impossible if you have to be civil to your host's children, or take an interest in the garden. Many hotels now have swimming pools and this is a convenient relaxational form of exercise. (Wet trunks travel well in a polythene bag!)

Ring up home twice a week and if you ring the office get them to ring your home to say that you are in good order. Letters are a poor way to communicate as they tend not to arrive.

The protected diet or the regular consumption of entro-vioform is not advocated, and generally if the natives can drink the water so can the visitor. However, a modest travelling medicine chest including aspirin, sleeping pills, gut-rot mixture and antibiotics is a good investment.

I hope that a word of warning about girls in night clubs will not be taken amiss. We see a modest trickle of senior men with guilty consciences, who have 'fallen' while in foreign parts, often celebrating a successful deal. If such activity is essential or desirable, and both could be the case, an old fashioned sheath or protective gives a fair degree of protection. It is a safe rule to remember that you cannot possibly be the only man to have had this relationship. If there is the slightest doubt, it is essential to seek medical advice before running any risk of infecting one's wife. Fatigue is a good excuse for delay, but not for avoiding treatment.

Further travel 'within the trip' should be just as carefully scheduled as for the outward and inward journeys and the same rules observed if there is any shift of time base. It is false economy to try and save a working day by flying at night from appointment to appointment.

Regular travellers should try to take their wives with them for at least one trip a year. Being accompanied by a wife makes for quite a different sort of trip, even if she has to amuse herself during the day.

Returning home

Getting back is always an anticlimax and much more tiring than going away. One is or tends to be exhausted and there is no longer the morale boosting challenge of the trip itself.

Exactly the same rules should be observed for the return trip and if it is possible to build in a short holiday in a congenial place, a stopover in a

Mediterranean villa or a couple of days with one's wife in a continental capital, this is desirable, but not always practicable. However, it is essential that the traveller gets adequate time off to re-acclimatize, recover and catch up with the family.

It is easy if the return is planned for Friday evening, but less easy mid-week. Sometimes half a day in the office may help with the debriefing, but it is probably better to have papers and secretary sent home to work in peace and away from the 'phone.

All these travel rules can be broken in the short term and by the young who are much more resilient. But if an individual is to remain effective and not get overtired, it must be realized that travel is much more demanding than normal work. It is a management responsibility to see that regular travellers are not exploited and that older travellers, those over 55, do it gracefully and gently. Individuals who are away a lot should be given extra holidays to compensate not only for fatigue, but also for family separation. The only trouble here is that the family will want to travel and father will be happy at home.

Effect on the family

There is no doubt that like many sailors' families, a number of business marriages survive better because of the regular absence of father, but in the main, the traveller's family has a thin time without him. As it affects domestic life, our current cultural behaviour pattern does depend on at least a minimum of shared activity between husband, wife and children. Continual absence, particularly over weekends, imposes a considerable strain on family ties. The wife left with young children finds the going hard and the evenings long, with no-one to commiserate with her about the awfulness of the day. The wife with no children has to look for outside interests.

It is in practice very difficult to catch up and patch up on the time lost by frequent overseas trips. Experience not shared tends to be experience or time lost. Families are not really interested in what happened in Bangkok airport and all father wants to do is sleep, not to hear about the village show or mother's headaches.

Children tend to survive into adolescence, but as this progresses, there may be problems, particularly now with drink, drugs and pregnancy. A very senior vice-president of an internation corporation with a flair for selling, a passion for international negotiation and a seemingly first class marriage, was suddenly faced with a 17 year old daughter with anorexia nervosa (psychogenic refusal to eat). The absentee father had certainly contributed to this breakdown.

Wives of businessmen seem to have a thin time anyway; wives of travellers have to make a lot of adjustments to remain sane and sensible. Talking to the experienced ones, they make the following points. Allow father to 'phone home frequently and, if he contacts the office, get them to pass on extra messages; this can also be two-way. In addition, some senior person should take the trouble to ring up home periodically and make sure that all is well. Wives stuck in the country can be in difficulty without a man to deal with crises or do heavy work. Give extra holidays to make up for absence and, as far as possible, older couples should try to arrange relaxational pursuits that are shared rather than done separately. Wives should be encouraged to travel when possible and make at least one trip a year. One European managing director of an American drug company insists on taking his wife on all trips lasting more than 2-3 days. As had already been suggested, senior and more affluent executives often find it sensible to have their wives meet them for a day or two at some congenial place on the way back. And those with Mediterranean villas find it possible to stay there surprisingly often.

At an export conference a year or two ago the wife of a more junior executive made a couple of good minor points. 'Please', she said, 'could we have a modest extra allowance for tropical suits and extra luggage', which airlines tend to destroy with monotonous efficiency.

On the whole, wives should be encouraged to participate in the 'life of the firm', to know what is going on and to be able to discuss her husband's problems with him. Frequent travel absences make this problem more acute and participation may help it to be more manageable and easier for the company to keep in touch with her.

NINE

Sleep

Sleep is precious enough to merit a section to itself. Some people are lucky in being able to put their heads on any pillow and sink like a stone. Others are even luckier and can additionally nod off in odd places and for short periods. The rest of us have varying degrees of difficulty in getting to and staying asleep. Others may find it hard to get enough of the right quality of sleep, especially when under pressure.

The importance of sleep

Physiologically sleep is a fascinating and, perhaps surprisingly, not an entirely understood occurrence. We do not know, for instance, whether sleep is imposed on wakefulness or *vice versa*. This may sound an odd protestation of professional ignorance, but if one looks firstly at animals in the wild, many of them only become active when they need food. Having fed, they often remain quiescent for several days. Other animals, particularly the herbivors, have a different pattern as they are continuous feeders.

Secondly, human young, and indeed the young of other species, when not eating, spend most of their time asleep. Thus, there is a case for suggesting that wakefulness is imposed, by need, on sleep.

Sleep is essential for short-term repair and maintenance of body tissues and the recharging of the energy batteries. To achieve this, during the sleep period, there is a 'shut down' of the energy consuming body processes. Thus, blood pressure, pulse, and respiration rate drop, digestion slows down and so too does kidney and other organ activity. The control of all this is through the brain and under the 24-hour governor system, which is responsible for circadian rhythm, ie much of the slow down happens even if the subject is awake.

Without enough sleep the subject 'feels tired' and is increasingly unable to function effectively, and after a certain period of sleep deprivation there is more or less total disintegration of effective functioning. This can be regarded as acute or short-term fatigue. More important is the longer-term fatigue, which is not so directly related to sleep loss, but arises from over-involvement and lack of holidays and recreational breaks. Thus, we need enough sleep within the 24-hour period and also, particularly with increasing age, adequate remissions for a more general recharging or toning up to take place.

Interestingly, on holiday, although people differ in their needs and behaviour, there is firstly, extra sleep and, secondly, rather peaceful, quite different and non-work related activities. It would appear that the work-related batteries get recharged so that normal life can be resumed with more zest. From clinical experience, it is found that older people take longer to recharge or bounce back, and part of their survival kit should include the discipline of not getting overtired in a way that they could, say, five years earlier. They perform much better if they keep on an even keel rather than oscillating between peaks and valleys of fatigue. All this also reinforces the need for and the value of relaxational pursuits, particularly those with a physical content. Sleep following exercise seems somehow to be more rewarding than that after a normally harassing day. A famous doctor once observed that exercise was the finest cure for anxiety. After an active day in the open air, it is almost impossible to keep awake no matter how tired one is. For similar reasons, a brisk walk before going to bed helps blow away the day's cobwebs. And a fairly lively dog helps to enforce the discipline. A slow stroll with a snuffling peke is of little good.

Although individuals vary considerably as to their sleep requirements, the amount of sleep each person requires remains remarkably constant. Lucky is the person who can get by with five hours and perhaps unlucky the one who needs eight. Sleep can be banked short term. Thus over a week or five working days a sleep overdraft can be run up and then paid off by extra sleep over the weekend.

Dreaming and discharge of tension

There is still some disagreement and confusion amongst the experts about the importance of dreaming. Some people clearly dream more than others or, at least, are more conscious of their dreams even though these may be harmful or frightening. Certain types of dream do give the psychiatrist some insight into what is on the patient's mind and how this tends to work. Although a fairly liberal dose of symbolism is needed to interpret some of the 'dream-world' happenings.

Whether or not dreams reach conscious memory, there is no doubt that during sleep a good deal of spontaneous rambling about goes on in various parts of the brain. It would appear that there is a need to discharge tension and perhaps regain balance. Current anxieties may often be reflected in the dreams and some people have a constantly recurring dream pattern. All this is quite normal.

Some of the objection held by a number of doctors to the regular use of sleeping pills is based on the suggestion that hypnotic pills, particularly inhibit the more active of the two types of sleep. (During normal sleep there are periods of subconscious activity and periods of rapid eye movements). It is suggested that damping this down stops necessary brain discharge with possible mildly harmful effects and reduction of the restorative value of the sleep period. The evidence for this is a bit thin and it has always been my view that no sleep is far worse than the lack of this type of sleep. Thus sleeping pills are strongly advocated by me.

Factors inhibiting sleep

Of course, the critical thing about sleep is getting to and staying there and here again people differ enormously in their rates and abilities. It appears that there is a gradual reduction of the sensory and stimulating input into the brain. As all activity ceases the sleep centre takes over and as it were switches off the cerebral cortex. All this is set in train by the relaxational ritual or habit pattern of going to bed. Stimulation is reduced and tranquillity sought after. Hence the warm bath, hot drink, beguiling book, comfortable bed, quiet room, etc.

Clearly then, and dependent on individual sensitivity, anything that interrupts this pattern will interfere with sleep. The two main factors which do this are either unfamiliar surroundings, which may include noise and bed, and anxiety. The first being largely external and the second self-generated. In either case the input is such that the brain cannot switch off and sleep is prevented or, and this is just as common, initial fatigue may be enough to get one to sleep but later on anxiety, or whatever it is, takes over and sleep is interrupted.

The sort of fugue state that anxiety seems to produce, is a good example of this. A simple set of ideas, often unimportant in themselves, seems to go round and round and keep one awake. The trick is to try and break the vicious circle, but this is easier said than done, particularly as one is reluctant to really wake up and perhaps risk disturbing one's partner. Counting sheep is the traditional way of trying to deal with this and a better variant, suggested by a colleague, Dr R. Romanis, is names. Start with A, or any other letter in the alphabet and try to think of five or ten girls and boys names beginning with the letter. In one's fuddled, semi-sleepy state, it is not as easy as it sounds, but it does take the mind off the fugue.

Obviously too, any disability, like pain, itchy skin, indigestion, etc, gets worse when there is nothing else to do but lie awake and think about it. Heart beat becomes prominent and the quite normal irregularities alarmingly noticeable. Pain is best dealt with by pain killers like Codeine and anxiety with tranquillizers. If this does not work it is probably sensible to wake up properly and do something different like going to the loo, making a cup of tea or reading for a while.

Aids to sleeping

Sleeping pills can be particularly useful when one expects not to sleep, eg when travelling or in unfamiliar places. Additionally, they may be kept by the bed so that if one is not asleep in about an hour a pill may be taken. The fact that they are there, in case needed, tends to limit there use. If one has a run of bad nights, it is sensible to take pills for at least a couple of nights running, to break the circle and get back on to an even keel. Some people are lucky enough never to need pills and others are frightened of becoming addicted or dependent on them. This is a legitimate fear, except that sleep results from a series of habits or conditioned reflexes and if a pill helps this along, it is far better than not sleeping and being continuously below par.

There are now such a wide range of pills to choose from and the changes can always be rung so that the dangers are minimal. The main danger comes from less-balanced people using an overdose for a suicide attempt. Pills come in all sorts of 'shapes and sizes', quick and slow acting and long and short lasting. It is sensible to experiment a little and find the most suitable.

A moderately recent introduction is a new type of drug which does not 'paralyse' the whole brain as does alcohol and the barbiturate hypnotics, but seems to have the capacity to switch off the central cortex and stop things buzzing around. These drugs, of which Mogadon is the best example, have the great advantage of being very safe in that even large overdoses are not dangerous.

There are a few unfortunate people who never sleep well or enough and they have to learn, having got their quota of sleep, to remain reasonably reposed and relaxed until getting up time. They will tell you how boring this is, but they do have to guard against using up some of the energy they will need during the day.

Marriages can be wrecked by snoring and doctors are sadly bad about dealing with it. It is always worth starting with one of the few experts who have taken an interest in the problem. With luck there may be a simple physical reason like a blocked nose. Otherwise pride must be shelved and decisions made to use earplugs or even separate rooms. Sleep is too precious to do without.

Sleep presents different problems as age advances. It seems to get lighter, more easily disturbed and needed in shorter periods. If necessary, this should be admitted and certainly in retirement arrangements made for an afternoon or early evening sleep. It seems likely that we would all be much better if we could divide the day more evenly by an extra sleep after lunch. One professor had a camp bed put out in his office after lunch and the whole department kept quiet until he was wakened at 1.55.

In fact, there is a very good physiological case for the cat-nap before the evening engagement and also to help older people keep awake and participate after supper. Similarly the older early waker can get up and potter, especially in the summer, knowing that he will catch up later.

Because older people tend inevitably to disturb each other increasingly and for a variety of reasons, the old-fashioned pot under the bed is less disturbing than putting lights on in the corridor. It is expedient not to be too proud about separate beds and later separate rooms. Again the need for both to get adequate sleep should be the overriding factor.

A last word about relaxation and aids to sleeping. It should by now be clear that the borderline between sleep and complete relaxation is fairly narrow. Thus, in the absence of true sleep, relaxation can be very restorative. There are a number of systems of relaxation from Yoga to transcendental meditation, and there are also teachers of and classes for learning to relax. Generally tense and highly strung people can derive great benefit from such instruction. Busy people can similarly learn to benefit from 20 minutes on the sofa or in the back of the car. There are also gimmicks for sleeping and relaxation ranging from wires connecting hands to feet, to stop vital energy ebbing away, to electromagnetic waistcoats and sleeping in the line of magnetism. As they are all harmless, anything that works is entirely legitimate.

TEN

Living with a coronary

One of the first articles I wrote for *The Director* was called 'When a Coronary can be a Blessing'. Needless to say, the title alone was criticized by the medical establishment. The burden of that particular article was that if a man was lucky enough to have had a mild coronary and then to have learnt from it, he should benefit mentally and physically from the experience. After all, it has always been respectable to profit from one's mistakes.

Shortly after this, on a visit to a medical colleague who advised a number of senior executives, I found him 'picking up the pieces' for someone who had been grossly mishandled by the hospital and his GP. The patient was immensely gloomy because all they had done was to tell him the things he could not do, which is the usual medical approach. 'Take it easy, don't strain yourself, in fact, abandon hope and wrap up in cotton wool.'

Over the years, doctors have been responsible, because they want to appear kind and cautious, for producing hundreds of unnecessary invalids. The body, in my view, is well able to look after itself. It will very soon let its owner know if something cannot be done. There is very little hard evidence for many chronic disabilities that effort makes the situation worse. Indeed, we know increasingly that we must positively struggle to maintain and redevelop the strength of weakened muscles and the movement of stiff joints. The heart is no exception to this rule.

Sudden attack

The man whose stress reaction takes the form of coronary artery atherosclerosis is, on the whole, unlucky, particularly if he does not attend for presymptomatic diagnosis. Other equally stressed men may get a duodenal ulcer or migraine. In either and many other cases, the symptoms ring a loud and clear bell which draws attention and demands avoiding action. The coronary, on the other hand, creeps silently up and strikes as it were from behind. The harm has been done without any previous danger signs.

As explained in Part One, coronary heart disease is a process in which, for a variety of reasons, the blood vessels to the heart muscle, coronary arteries, get narrowed by disease and finally blocked by a blood clot. Though the actual blockage is sudden, painful, dramatic and frightening, it is the result of a long-standing and gradual process which in practical terms is more important than the event, unexpected though this may be.

Coronary thrombosis is the commonest cause of sudden death and about a third are fatal, either immediately or within a week or so. Modern intensive care units have put up the survival rate a little, but there is now some doubt as to their real value. Contrary to popular belief, coronaries occur more or less evenly over the 24 hours. One hears about the dramatic cases on golf courses or at meetings and not about the ones at home and in bed. The other encouraging thing is, of course, the considerable powers of survival and recovery shown by some people. Given this in the initial stages, surgery may help later by pleating flabby muscle, improving blood supply by arterial grafting and possibly electronic pacemakers.

Outlook and attitude

The outlook, or as doctors say, the prognosis following a heart attack, depends on a number of factors. Obviously and firstly, on how extensive the thrombosis was and how much functional heart muscle is left. Secondly, on the state of the blood supply to this muscle and the general degree of cardiovascular disease. Thirdly, as we have already stressed, the physical state of the patient and his heart muscle. Muscle in good training has great powers of standing up to the insult of the thrombosis.

Fourthly, and usually critically in terms of the quality of survival, is the attitude of mind of the patient and his wife. As a major part of the readjustment, he must discover what it was in his behaviour pattern that produced the attack and then readjust happily to avoid it. This will probably involve an agonizing reappraisal of aspirations and attributes.

Rehabilitation

The concern here is to discuss mental (in outline) and physical rehabilitation and not to get involved in technical detail. Rehabilitation should start the moment the patient gets into hospital or into medical care at home. (A high proportion of coronaries can be treated perfectly well at home, perhaps with a nurse for a week or so.) The point, however, is to restore morale to patient and wife immediately. After all, the patient is still alive and there is every reason to believe that he will not only recover but get back to full function. Statistics show that the great majority of 'sedentary' coronary patients get back to their original work. A number of studies have shown the benefit of sympathetic psychological handling of both patients − husband and wife. Having dealt with the shock they are then given an active survival philosophy. A coronary survived is neither a death sentence nor condemnation to permanent invalidism. The patient must be encouraged to *do* things and not given lists of restrictions.

Because it was thought that damaged heart muscle took three months to become hard scar tissue, the tradition used to be three months protected existence with about a month of it in bed. Very serious coronaries apart, it is now known that there is no hard evidence that early activation, getting out of bed, etc, does any harm. We want to avoid ending up with a flabby wreck that has to be dragged back to fitness. Early activation, early discharge from hospital and intensive but controlled physical rehabilitation should be the aim and is increasingly recommended. There are now special physical rehabilitation courses for post-coronary patients and admirable they are. The key is graded exercise leading to reasonable exertion in six months or so. This includes gentle running, golf, swimming, anything which gradually makes the heart earn its keep and develop new blood vessels in response to the demands of training. In ordinary social terms the patient should aim at a little more every day. Climbing stairs is good training and can be done at home on a cold wet day. Too little activity is more dangerous than too much.

Obviously doctors must deal with any predisposing causes and survival may well depend on not slipping back into bad habits. Weight must be ruthlessly dealt with, probably all smoking stopped, blood pressure and cholesterol treated and so on. Remember that alcohol dilates blood vessels and is usually encouraged in modest amounts. This latter will produce a dramatic improvement in well-being and is part of the potential blessing. It is also a practical demonstration of the philosophy of activity and graded progress as an aid to banishing the inevitable anxiety about the future.

As already said, coronary heart disease is a process and the outlook can only depend on what is left and how generalized the disease is. To a degree, the younger the better, but given proper behaviour many of the processes can be reversed and the circulation improved. Up to recently, it was not uncommon for a post-coronary patient to be given anticoagulant treatment, sometimes for years. This was to try and stop the blood clotting again in the damaged arteries. It was inconvenient treatment and there is little statistical evidence as to its value.

Rules for survival

It used to be said that every six months survived halved the chances of recurrence. Certainly after a year, the outlook is usually excellent, provided remedial action is one hundred per cent. So after four or five years the event can largely be forgotten.

The main aim, however, should be to analyse what in the whole life situation produced the coronary. Indulgences like smoking and physical sloth apart, what stresses and tensions drove the man to this state? There may have been personality clashes, uncongenial work, too much pressure, aspiration outstepping attributes and so on. Survival depends on redeploying the patient in a less pressurized life pattern, if necessary at a lower level.

The ground rules of the survival game are clearly stated: calm down, keep fit and survive; press on regardless and die. Obviously though, because of the personality factors which motivated the attack, the calming down is easier to preach than to achieve. It must be a real, happily accepted reappraisal and not a resentful one. If the man remains hankering after his mis-spent past he will not really reduce the internal tension. As already implied, a psychiatric reassessment can be very helpful in coming to terms with the modified personality. In my medical utopia, the psychiatrist and the physical training expert are the leaders of the rehabilitation team.

In fact, if all this can be reasonably achieved, the individual will be living within his limitations and far happier for it. Following mild to moderate coronaries almost normal physical activity can be regained and there is everything to play for. Resist all attempts to be turned into an invalid. 'Use your heart until it hurts' and you won't come to any harm. This includes sex, which is to be treated like all other physical activity. I never put a physical restriction on a patient unless I know it will be harmful. Anything that the body can be trained to do without too much revolt is desirable. It is wise to start off with rather modest achievement and work targets but to say that the backwater is not permanent. The situation should be reviewed annually with a view to permitting sailing in deeper waters.

There is a major role for wives in all this. Firstly, they must encourage optimism without cossetting. Secondly, they must enforce dietary, physical and other discipline. Thirdly, they must make it quite clear that they would rather have a live, peaceful husband than be the widow of a failed tycoon, because a coronary before retirement is a failure to balance the personality-environment equation.

We have scores of patients, many of them chairmen and other senior people, others much more junior, who are now well into their seventies, years after a coronary. They have learnt the lesson and seen the light and they remain under very regular maintenance so that the earliest deviation can be picked up.

ELEVEN
The Quality of Marriage

Because of our 'whole man' approach to the causes of 'dis-ease', we have always been interested in domestic and family life. Additionally, for a long time, my personal concern has been the problems of relationships, the glue that is required to make people stick together and often the rather inadequate reasons for continuing a marriage. It has always seemed sad that such a high proportion of relationships rub along, without there being much in it for either participant, ie the impression is that the quality of marriage tends to be poor.

Domestic stress

At The Institute of Directors when we started analysing the main causes of stress in 1964, we soon found that nearly as much came from home as did from work. Indeed, it was difficult to escape the view stated earlier, that executives understood the work situation rather better than they did the domestic one, which tended to be taken for granted and given inadequate nourishment. Equally, as already mentioned, executives tend to be bad at people and good at things. There is, however, more to this situation than just the executive's problem. In all justice we need also to look at 'what is in it for the wife'. Her side of the penny is, in medical and community terms, just as important as his. But in a masculine world, she tends to be somewhat neglected.

When we started the Medical Research Unit in 1958, there was some anxiety about the claims rate of the Institute of Director's very large BUPA group. When asked about this, I was overjoyed because I thought that an analysis of the claims experience would bring to light all I needed to know about 'directors' diseases'. With expert epidemiological advice, we set up a very detailed investigation to analyse the IOD group experience and compare it with a non-business control group. Sadly, and for technical reasons connected with the lack of a coherent diagnostic policy in certification, we got little of direct medical interest out of all this, but we did discover something about the family health pattern.

It soon became apparent that the claims rate for wives and children was appreciably higher in the directors than in the control group. The wives it appeared (here I am interpreting freely) were an unhappy lot who paraded up and down Harley Street calling for, in psychosomatic terms, help for their dis-ease. Because of the nature of disease and symptom-oriented medicine, they were given endless operations and expensive treatments. The situation was inescapably like the eminent specialist in Shaw's *The Doctor's Dilemma* who removed the 'nuciform sac' at great profit to himself.

Currently in our rather too rapid for comfort social evolution, we are going through a period of change and instability which is reflected in a lack of understanding and failure of communication between parents and children. This, in turn, appears to have contributed to or increased the natural rebeliousness and aggression that goes with adolescence, much of which probably goes back to poor or second rate marital and domestic relationships. Marriage often is something which tends to be taken as a usual course of action and embarked on with inadequate thought and preparation. Similarly, it is not realized how difficult good relationships really are and what is required to foster them.

Within a possible rather low quality marriage, mother tends to get rather taken for granted and expected to provide a rather demanding service for which she gets scant reward. Shut any father up for a week with a demanding three-year-old child, and he is likely to be pretty frayed and demented at the end of the exercise. Yet he expects his wife to put up with this day-in and day-out, and to come up smiling with a splendid supper as he crawls exhausted off the commuter express, perhaps smelling slightly of drink.

It appears, though, that women largely have themselves to blame for accepting this rather 'dog's body' role. It is recommended that they take a much more demanding line and get a lot more husband participation in the home life. The liberation of women is not really related to the survival of the brassiere, but it does concern their emotional needs in more equal relationships.

Having said this and wanting to pass on later to a brief consideration of what constitutes a good relationship, these comments must be qualified with the realization that this is known to be a particularly dangerous field for generalization. The spectrum of satisfaction in human behaviour is so wide that anything will seemingly go for a minority of people. Looking round one's own social circle, it is easy to see something of the range. The simplest type of relationship to criticize is the dependent one in which a dominant partner, often a woman, seems to henpeck a rather poor little husband. The latter never seems to stand up for himself and might even enjoy being trampled on. The probability is that if he was liberated from this seeming dominance, he would be lost and almost incapable of independent existence.

Such a man may himself be dominant at work and put up with being second fiddle at home. Although there may be large sado-masochistic elements in the relationship, the assumption is that there is enough in it for both of them to make it worthwhile. And this is the key to the relationship situation: there must be enough in it for both of them, which means that both must contribute to and nurture the relationship to make it worthwhile.

Poor relationships

One of the main problem areas about relationships appears to be the particular difficulties of intelligent and demanding people. Just as it is necessary to perceive conflict to be stressed, ie the simple minded take life as it comes without much question, so intelligent and involved people are either much more demanding in what they want out of relationships or do not seem to have much time for them.

Taking this even further, it may be pointed out that there are many outstanding people (who are themselves in a minority) be they creative artists, scientists, politicians or businessmen, who tend neither to have time for good relationships nor to be good at them. One of the things that happens is that they get so involved in and identified with their main stream activity, that there is not room for anything else. Additionally, their mental lives and emotional development becomes so unbalanced that they tend also to have rather bad and naive judgements about areas remote from their expertise.

However, life does tend to be made easier for them because of the way in which their charisma and pre-eminence attracts a 'fan club', which makes for a series of short-term adoring relationships which break up because they are not really important to the 'leader', and in any case he is reluctant to contribute anything to them. Some businessmen fall into this category, partly because they may be outstandingly good at their jobs and partly because of the commitment they are making to the development of their careers. Business is a particularly demanding life, although highly satisfying and rewarding, because it involves long hours, endless crises, developing contacts, willingness to travel and be available, and so on. These activities being both demanding and satisfying really leave neither time nor energy for anything else, including a marital relationship requiring at least some input and availability from the man.

Over the years I have got into mild trouble by saying that men in this group would be better off with a competent housekeeper and an occasional mistress rather than a wife. There is always a howl of outrage from the downtrodden wife who sees herself officially displaced by the 'girlfriend', who may already exist. But the main point here is that these people should *never have got married* in the first place. If they have a wife and family, they have a real responsibility to give up enough of their work to make a reasonable commitment to the marriage.

The much more common type of poor relationship is the one in which boredom seems to predominate and there really is not enough in it for either party. Equally it is not bad enough to produce a crisis so it goes rubbing along at rather a low level and producing what seems to be a low-quality personal existence. This is, of course, the sort of situation which is easily disrupted by the sudden appearance of a more stimulating alternative, the bright girlfriend or the gay young man at the cocktail party.

It seems that some business marriages tend to come into both these last two categories. The man takes it all rather for granted, pays the bills and expects to be well looked after. His wife gets used to providing a service and getting rather little satisfaction in return and they are likely to have a decreasing amount in common particularly when the children have grown up.

It seems that before it happens a lot more thought should be given to what marriage is all about, why it is being undertaken and what might be in it for both parties. It is deplorable that people tend to get married early before they know what they want, what sort of people they want to be and what life is all about. It is now so perfectly possible and desirable to sample life together before marriage, that it would seem sensible to do so. At least, now, relatively few people start marriage with the appalling sexual ignorance and inexperience that burdened the great middle class up to quite recently.

However if, rightly or wrongly, a marriage with children has been established, the couple owe it to the children to make it a good one. And here the wife has got to start much earlier in the relationship, in getting a better bargain and greater commitment from her spouse. He must not be allowed to develop the habit of treating his home as a hotel and buying his way out of emotional involvement with expensive presents.

The right partner

The first problem inevitably is who to marry, and although this tends to be fortuitously related to social and other contacts, the dice can be loaded against the choice by the woman, particularly, being incompatible with the demands of her husband's career. Professor Ray Pahl of the University of Kent has done some sociological study in this area, on executive family patterns. It became apparent to him that the best wife for an executive was a competent secretary who, because she had been through part of the mill, would at least understand his life and its problems. A more academic or social person would resent his involvement and the mobility involved. This situation is likely to improve, as more young girls take on serious jobs to get away from home and become self-supporting.

Social class can present problems which have already been mentioned. If the two partners do not grow at the same rate, the wife becomes miserable and feels increasingly dis-eased by the type of environment she is asked to inhabit. The best solution to this incompatibility seems to be a civilized divorce and a fresh start. A relatively large number of successful executives have had to do this.

Marriages, in my view, are much more likely to succeed if they start from maturity and possibly even from previous experience. They start off by meaning so much more and because of this extract enough commitment to make them work.

Having looked at the difficult ones, it is fair to admit that obviously a high proportion of business marriages rub along reasonably well and both participants are not dissatisfied, but it is surprising how few people give an affirmative answer to our question: has your marriage been as happy as you would have liked?

Child management

However, particularly if the right balance has not been struck, the next set of problems may well arise from the teenage children. Parents are suddenly confronted with a problem area which they do not understand and to which their lack of involvement is clearly a contributory factor. The guilt that goes with this does not make dealing with the situation any easier. And, in any case, it can be a very difficult situation for even the most enlightened and dedicated parents.

In addition, and without overt problems, it is not fair (and mothers constantly complain about this) to leave all or most of child management to mother. Father does no disciplining, comes home and 'spoils' and tends to leave mother out on a limb as rather a dragon. It is essential that as far as possible father should fully participate in all aspects of rearing his children. Older parents, who marry later, are far better at this because the children somehow seem to mean so much more, ie they take higher priority. In any case, father might have a bit more time and energy by then.

The under-occupied wife

If this hazard is survived, the next one is: what happens as they both get older? By now, mother may be used to leading her own life and may have her own involvements, or she may be becoming bored, isolated and perhaps in order to justify her existence, a bit too obsessed with being a housewife. In other words running the home becomes an end in itself and anything that interferes with it is resented and complained about. And this very much includes attempts to use the house as a home, muck it up a bit, or bring people in unexpectedly, etc. This type of person can be very trying to live with. They also tend to find it difficult to establish adult relationships with their children, because they want some one to be both dependent and 'obedient' and will not accept that they have grown up.

Women who drift in this direction may have started life with professional or semi-professional skills, but as the drift progresses they become reluctant to get back into the world, re-use their skills and take up jobs or activities which will get them back into circulation. One particular case was that of the rather pathetic, childless wife to a great tycoon who used only to go back to his semi-baronial home for a short weekend. Sunday appeared to be taken up with church and a board meeting, because the factory was up the road from his house. When asked what she did all day, she replied 'I do the flowers'. Rather unkindly, I asked 'Why?', as her husband was away all week. In fact, she was a tragically unhappy person and, although she had everything material she wanted, her life was empty. Interestingly, she died several years before her husband.

It is easy to see how this type of person becomes dis-eased, suffers from all sorts of aches and pains and ceases to be much fun to live with. But, as mentioned previously, many wives of businessmen get the worst end of the deal and very little job satisfaction out of being married to 'him'. It is surprising how seldom, in marriages that have rubbed along without much friction, the husband looks objectively at his wife's life and tries to see what is in it for her. One of the things he can be encouraged to do is to persuade her, as the children grow up, to get back into the widest possible circulation. This is discussed further in the next section on retirement.

Relationships in the grown-up family

Another area of neglect and difficulty is that of the two-way relationship between parents and grown-up or adult-age children. Both sides find it very difficult to establish free adult, rather than dependent parent-child, relationships. Clearly it is better for the community, and very much part of our cultural pattern, that families should remain coherent. Under this code of behaviour, children are on the whole expected to look after their aged parents who in turn help by being active and efficient grandparents.

But there is nothing inevitable about this and biologically the young go out into the world to establish their own identity. This is what parents, particularly mothers, resent about their children; they disapprove of the identity which rightly or wrongly their young establish. This in turn, makes the children resentful of their parents, so that contact becomes a burden and not a joy. There is also a type of mother who specializes in being anxious about her grandchildren and the way in which they are brought up.

When I remarried, my second wife thought I was far too tolerant of my student children and ought to extract more respect and obedience, etc. It seems to me that after a certain time parents are largely at the receiving end and should stop trying to interfere or alter. A better adult relationship is likely to result. Another point is that children, to a degree, while resenting the way they are treated by their parents, are reluctant to complain. To a considerable degree, particularly with advancing age, the parents are dependent so that the young can and could call much more of their own tune. This stops them getting irritated and makes for a better relationship; one major row is better than constant bickering and friction.

Diverging interests

A fascinating thought about marriage relationships is either why they should not be worse than they sometimes are or why, for the same reasons, marriages ever survive at all. (The answer to this may well be partly lack of incentive to change and lack of guts so to do). The point here is that people who marry under the age of 25 are inevitably relatively immature. It is fairly unclear what their interests, talents and requirements might come to be. The chances are at least equal that they will develop in different rather than the same directions, and twenty years later there may well not be enough glue to hold the relationship together.

Provided no-one suffers too much, I take the view that it is better with goodwill and in a civilized way, to stop unsatisfactory marriages, rather than continue them in a state of nagging acquiescence.

Sharing interests

One of the most interesting problems about business marriage in particular, is what do you talk to your wife about? There is a school of thought which never takes the office home. Thus the wife knows and understands little about what her husband does or who he does it with. This attitude may be splendid in theory, and it tends to get mixed up with 'Oh, I don't want to bore her with that', but if work is excluded as a topic of conversation, what is there left to talk about?

It seems fairly certain that reasonably successful marriages depend on building bridges and establishing common ground. As work fills so much of the businessman's life, and as he is on the whole short of people to talk to about himself and his problems, it is desirable that he should talk to his wife, in confidence, about what is happening in his world. The chances are high that not only will she be a sounding board and a shoulder to lean on, but also that her comments might help. In addition, if he is surrounded by 'yes' men, she might even cut him down to size. I am strongly in favour of sharing as much experience as possible, though what happens when husband and wife work in the same organization, or run it together, I am not sure, but suspect that it is dangerous. What on earth do they talk about except work?

One of the problems of travel, provided that it is not a means of escaping, is that separation is experience not shared. If a man is away from home for a month at a time, which is not uncommon, his wife has to lead her own life and deal with her problems. When he gets back, she is no more interested in what happened in Singapore, indeed, she may be mildly suspicious of what might have happened with the dusky maidens, than he is in the mores of village life.

Related to these problem areas is the extent to which the wife wants to participate in her husband's business activities. This involves entertaining, visiting the office and getting to know the people there, sometimes travel and generally picking up the bits. A small scale questionnaire was done several years ago and in this, a number of wives complained that they were neither encouraged nor given the opportunity to be 'part of the company'.

The classical example of this situation is, of course, the politician's wife; unless she is prepared for bazaar opening and political tittle tattle she is doomed to isolation. Unless she has strong alternative views, my firm advice to wives is to get tactfully involved. The business associates may be wildly boring, but at least you know what your husband is up to and can get him home a bit earlier.

Divorce

The perms on good and satisfying relationships are infinite. The trauma and stress that can be caused, both positively and negatively, by unsatisfactory relationships is extensive and not uncommon. Trying to help several senior executives over the divorce hurdle recently, it was obvious that their lives and doubtless those of the wives too, had been made miserable for years by incompatible and nagging marriages. There is no need to take sides to see that they are busy scratching each other and that it is time that goodwill is exercised to stop it. Even if bilateral goodwill cannot be achieved, unilateral separation is better than continuous misery, usually skilfully exploited by one party. I suspect that there is a reluctance to face what is thought likely to be the social opprobria of divorce, but having been through this myself, I can speak for the advantages of a fresh start.

Life is quite difficult enough without making it more so by perpetuating an unsatisfactory relationship. Life is for living, and it cannot be lived in a state of chronic misery. It is doubtful too, if the difficult party, usually said to be the wife, would in fact be any more unhappy if she was set up in a flat. At least only one person would then be miserable.

Clearly, if children are involved, the situation is more complicated and their needs must predominate until they are reasonably independent or emotionally secure. Here too, however, the opinion of the experts is changing. It used to be thought that two warring parents were *always* better than one. But there is now a feeling that there may be occasions where one stable parent provides a better base than two in constant conflict. Also it must be borne in mind that children who seldom show any sign may be both sensitive and perceptive about friction between their parents. Even if they are not present, they know about the rows and the incompatibility and it may scar them for life.

Improving relationships

Nothing I can write will make the difficulty of good interpersonal relationships, in marriage or within the company any easier, but by emphasizing and oversimplifying the problems, it is hoped that the following points have been made. Firstly that, on the whole, one is lucky if the 'good' just emerges; mostly it has to be sought after and nurtured. Secondly, and this is extremely important, if there is a problem, it must be dealt with and not allowed to fester. It must be dealt with first by admitting that it exists, second by defining it, third by looking at the options, which are determined by the personality of the participants, and fourth by doing something. Problems must be openly discussed and a solution agreed and stuck to.

Stress arises from the conflict of unsolved problems. Solution tends to come from grasping the nettle rather than pretending that there are no weeds in the garden.

One last plea needs to be made and this is once again to encourage women to drive a harder bargain in establishing a positive relationship and not being taken for granted as 'domestic provider'. Gloomy though the thought may be, they should also keep at the back of their minds, the realization that about a third of business wives will become widows before their husbands retire. If they learn some of the lessons outlined in this book, they can play a major role in reducing the odds against this happening to them. Further, women can help by encouraging, indeed demanding, sensible living to aid the growth of preventive medicine.

An area that can cause friction, resentment and anxiety is that of money. Husbands do not realize how undignified it is for a wife to have no money of her own and to be dependent on the housekeeping for her personal requirements.

Secrecy about income is a Victorian hangover, but it still persists, particularly in business circles. A recent survey showed that even today a high proportion of wives have no idea what their husbands either earn or receive as interest. All they get is the housekeeping money. How can a couple have a good relationship on the basis of this one sided dependancy?

Psychologically, there is a lot to be said for the joint bank account which overcomes much of this. To a degree, change in the right direction is occurring with the advent of the working wife. Earlier marriage with shared endeavour should make later secrecy much less tenable.

Another area of anxiety and ignorance is the problem of pensions and provision for the family in the not unlikely event of something happening to the husband. It is grossly unfair to leave all this to 'the reading of the will'. Contingency planning over resources right through life should be openly discussed and reviewed regularly. Such participation will make for much better long-term relationships.

TWELVE

The Woman Executive

Women who hold senior appointments in industry and commerce will probably deny that they are different from men or that they have different problems in holding down their jobs and meeting the ordinary challenges of business and domestic life and dealing with the men in their lives. From the contact I have had over the years with working women, I would not entirely agree with this. Although a married woman running a home, raising a family and then getting back into the world, has plenty of problems, which many of them appear to fail to solve adequately, the women executive or secretary, or factory worker for that matter, who does two jobs and does them well, has to be both tough and well organized to survive without too much conflict.

It is an interesting but fruitless speculation to consider why women, with their greater numbers and powers of survival, have not in fact made a greater contribution as community leaders, in any one of a number of fields. Probably it is because they have been systematically conned by men into being active mothers and housewives. Mostly they accept this as expected of them, but apart from actually producing and breastfeeding babies, there is no inherent reason why mother should not bring home the bacon and father change the nappies. Or is there? Are both of them in fact not capable of this role reversal? I do not know, but it is surprising that more women do not try for less domestic subservience, and in this book, several pleas are made for more equal relationships within marriage.

The dual role

The Institute of Directors has always had a small but appreciable proportion of women members and over the years attempts have been made, by questionnaire, to find out something about them. Unfortunately, a high proportion of them are relatively inactive directors of family firms. The rest are very hard working and far better organized than their menfolk. To hold down a job and run a home and family, requires a good set of priorities and the clear headedness to keep them sorted out. Also it occasionally means the willingness to give it all up, at least temporarily, to deal with a family crisis or look after a relative.

Women who survive in this dual role have to start by being fit and then to remain well by keeping in balance and avoiding fatigue and too much conflict. The chances are that to do this they have on the whole to be unusually stable emotionally, indeed perhaps a bit unemotional. Provided they can cope, they do not, in our limited experience, seem to have any extra problems and perhaps they are ultimately better off than the bored and lonely housewife who gets pain in her back when the children have left home.

Obviously, a woman in a man's world has advantages and disadvantages and she is quite entitled to exploit the former, but the ordinary sexual attractions of life, plus the added conflicts of home and career, etc, can impose a strain which has to be dealt with as objectively as possible. It seems that one of the main problems such women face is, that for a variety of reasons, women within organizations tend to be bad at dealing with each other. Secretaries tend not to like working for women and the supervisory woman tends not to be good at managing the girls. Obviously this is a generalization to which there are plenty of exceptions. Certainly, the Merchant Banking and Investment World is currently growing a crop of extremely bright and able young ladies and it will be interesting to see if they in fact go on and up, or after a few years drift back to suburbia.

Common hazards

Women in administrative roles obviously face all the hazards that men do, for example over-indulgence in alcohol, tobacco, work, lack of leisure. They probably have to devote more time, trouble and money to looking smart; they tend as a group to be more disciplined over diet and weight, but the few that fail in this do carry a greater social surcharge than say overweight or heavy-drinking men. As already noted, alcohol and nicotine do present hazardous slopes and the woman executive is well advised to be particularly careful about them.

Unfortunately, we do not have any mortality or morbidity figures relating to the differences between working and domestic women. As we have seen, women have a greater life expectancy and lower death rate at all ages than do men. I suspect, but cannot prove, that working women, particularly if they smoke heavily, do less well than those who stay at home. Certainly, a couple of coronaries in leading women in this group come to mind, but it must be added that anecdotal memory is profoundly unreliable statistically.

The unmarried career woman

Again without a great deal of experience, it seems that in many ways it is the unmarried career woman who has more problems than her married counterpart. Our society expects mature adults to pair off and mate like everyone else, and to be a bit suspicious about the few who do not. There seem to be three or four categories of unmarried people, and men, too, can be divided into the same groups.

The first and easiest category comprises reasonably attractive, mature and marriagable people who have objectively opted against marriage at least for the time being. They tend to be emotionally stable, may have extra-marital sexual associates, and tend to do well, without emotional conflict.

The second category comprises the frightened, the unattractive, the emotionally immature and rather inadequate people. They tend for all these reasons to be failures, but a few of them succeed, partly as an over compensation for their failure in other areas. Obviously this group does have emotional problems and the women more so than the men. In addition, and because of their emotional insecurity, they tend to go through crises either because they try too hard and fail or they get caught and get into a jam.

The third category is the small homosexual group, either overt and active, or sublimated and expressed by over-compensatory extrovert behaviour in other areas. It is probably easier (and again I am far from being an expert) for women to live a stable homosexual or lesbian life than it is for men. Perhaps this is because the relationships tend to be more stable and certainly it is made easier by a far greater toleration by society of women living together. Obviously this type of relationship or sublimation does produce emotional problems but they seem to get themselves dealt with, and those involved appear capable of living useful, secure and happy lives without undue breakdown.

The fourth category is the 'failed married' and comprises firstly those who have tried marriage with the result that it just has not worked out, with or without the production of children. Obviously, this produces severe conflicts which the individual does well to survive without too much scarring. The second subgroup is those who want to get married but cannot find the right partner or have left it all too late. Thus they need a good deal of insight to deal with their deprivation.

As a generalization, it seems likely that second marriages tend to be more successful and less conflict ridden than poor first ones. Both participants know what they are in for, they have presumably gone into it with their eyes open, and more determined to give and take enough to try and make it all work. Easy divorce seems to be the obvious answer, provided the children do not suffer unduly. (Incidentally, they tend to suffer more than is admitted from rowing parents and an unstable home.) There seems to be no point in perpetuating unhappy relationships for social reasons. People in this main category are likely to marry later in life, be more mature and make a greater success of it, if only because marriage has become so much more important and they have thought it out better.

The main worry in this area is the fate of the unmarried person, particularly the woman, when she retires. During her working life she has, to a degree, made up for the lack of domestic association and relationship by 'marrying her work', which also gives her an identity, association and income. When all this suddenly ceases at 60, five years earlier than for men, which in view of the mortality figures is totally irrational, she really is likely to be in trouble and a number of emotional chickens may come home to roost. This is when close family ties are immensely valuable because any retired person must have social and personal contacts.

Unfortunately many unmarried professional women have got into this state, because they are single and isolated and their retirement does then pose additional problems. They must get themselves into a situation where they at least live in proximity to other people and do things for them, so as to feel wanted. Otherwise they may become fiercely and neurotically independent and invent things to do, to disguise their loneliness. This group probably needs a lot of help and advice and we do not yet know the best answers for them.

General health problems

As far as general health is concerned, women face the same problems as men, but do have a few additional ones related to their reproductive cycles and systems. It is unfortunate in this respect that the great majority of doctors are men who are bored by and not really interested in women's rather unexciting gynaecological problems. Equally however, as women do not seem to trust each other they appear to prefer men to women doctors. Certainly the latter who take to gynaecology (women's diseases) tend to be better at the mechanical rather than the emotional side of their work.

Women do have a very complicated reproductive cycle, the monthly 'preparation for pregnancy' leading to menstruation; if, as is virtually always the case, there is no pregnancy, this provides plenty of opportunity for the participating organs and systems, including very much the psyche, to get out of adjustment and cause tension. Pregnancy, parturition and breastfeeding, which may occur two or three times during life, provide another series of changes and possible complications. Finally, the run-down of the reproductive system between 45 and 50 produces a further and difficult set of changes and need for adjustment.

Some gynaecological problems

This is not the place to write a 'woman's guide' to gynaecology, but simply to outline the areas of possible upset and make a plea for effective and understanding treatment. Firstly, however, one must make the general point that women, particularly as they get older, must observe all the health disciplines described for men. Regular exercise comes more easily to them because housework and shopping tends to be more active than being driven to the office and going up in the lift. However, women do need to watch their weight, avoid more than about five cigarettes a day, do exercises to remain supple and watch their appearance. Sadly, perhaps, men are allowed to run more overtly to seed, but women are in danger of being left behind or have their husband looking for alternative and more pleasurable ladies. Thus they have to take more trouble over remaining as attractive and lively as possible.

As far as pelvic disease is concerned, the womb, vagina and ovaries are liable to disease and malfunction. Vaginal infections, which need not be and seldom are strictly venereal, are boring, irritating and messy to treat. All one can do is to find a sympathetic doctor or clinic and peg away until cured. Some of these infections can be transferred to the marital partner and hence go backwards and forwards. Both will have to be treated.

Cancer of the womb and cervix are not uncommon and the cervical smear has now become as accepted as was mass chest radiography. Both smear clinics and the family-planning session provide a good opportunity to discuss minor problems. Any unusual bleeding, at any age, but particularly after the change of life (menopause), should be treated seriously. There are plenty of benign causes for this and include the benign womb tumour called a fibroid. Diagnosis is made by what is called 'dilation and currettage' or D & C. Under a light anaesthetic the neck of the womb is stretched to allow a scraping instrument to be introduced. The lining of the womb is then removed and examined under a microscope. Abortions are done in much the same way although now there are more sophisticated suction methods of evacuation.

Once the diagnosis has been made it may be necessary to surgically remove the womb. This is not a particularly serious operation and it does not impede future sexual activity. All that is being done is to remove a worn out and no longer needed piece of apparatus, but obviously, this does have emotional connotations and many women feel deprived and different after the operation. A man may find this difficult to understand, believing that it must give the woman advantages with no more monthly periods to cope with.

Particularly following several children, the womb may get a bit loose and tend to fall downwards and outwards. This is called a prolapse and is due to weakness of the pelvic and vaginal muscles. Surgical repair is successful, simple and again does not interfere with sex.

Painful periods, dysmenorrhea, is virtually unknown in non-western countries, where women are expected to get on with life without a fuss, and often to do hard physical work into the bargain. Victorian mothers used to brings their daughters up expecting their periods to be painful, just as they were taught that sex was something men did to them and which they tolerated for the sake of keeping their husbands happy and for having children. Times and attitudes have changed, women are equal and legitimately demanding sexual partners and painful periods less common. There are, of course, mechanical reasons for the pain, but most of this is due to emotional tension made worse by the swelling up and general tension produced by the cyclical hormonal changes at the end of the cycle. This is known as premenstrual tension and (to men) is a boring and mildly disabling condition. It can be dealt with, both symptomatically with hormones and painkillers and by dealing with the emotional conflicts etc. It should be totally unnecessary and discouraged to take to one's bed for a regular day or so off. It is an interesting piece of industrial experience that rest-rooms provided for women staff tend to get used in relation to their availability, ie if they are not provided many fewer people have to be sent home.

Having said this, one must also make the point that there are physical causes for painful periods and if these persist or fail to respond to simple analgesics, professional advice should be sought.

One further gynaecological word concerns any irregular vaginal bleeding, either between periods while still menstruating or after they have stopped, which, like all other bleeding, is a cause for immediate investigation. Most causes will be trivial and easily dealt with, but if they are more serious the sooner treatment is instigated the greater the chances of cure. Particularly with regard to gynaecological conditions, pain, bleeding, discharge or discomfort all merit treatment. 'Up with them the lady should not put'.

There is no doubt that 'the pill' has made it far easier and more reliable to have regular and normal sexual lives without fear of pregnancy. Although other mechanical contraceptive methods exist and work well if carefully used, the pill is by far the most acceptable to most people. It acts by interfering with the hormonal basis on which ovulation and fertilization occur, and to a degree this is interfering with the natural cycle. A recent large scale follow-up trial has demonstrated the safety of the pill, but it can have side effects and there are probably a few people who should not take it. There is also a choice of types of pill and the question of the right type is very much a matter of expert judgement. Pills should not just be handed out; they should be both tailored, supervised and monitored to the idiosyncracies of the individual.

Successful sexual activity makes life more satisfying for most people; failure to achieve this can be very stressful and a prime cause of guilt and anxiety. This is not the place to discuss these problems except to make the general point that if there is a problem it must be faced, admitted, brought into the open and discussed. Otherwise it may fester and cause a great deal of conflict and tension.

Similarly the inability to have children can be both a sorrow and a hardship in which it is difficult to avoid either apportioning blame or looking for scapegoats. Twenty years ago it was fashionable to blame all sterility or subfertility, on the woman. Now we know that not only are at least ten per cent of marriages sterile, but that the cause of the sterility can be on either partner, or indeed a mixture of both. This is again a matter for expert advice and investigation and much can be done to improve the chances. An important thing the expert can do is to tell the couple what the chances are and if they are hopeless or very borderline, much anxiety can be relieved by stopping hoping and trying too hard.

I am a protagonist of adoption and I have seen numerous happy families based on this. Often in borderline cases, adopting one child will relieve the tension and natural pregnancy may follow. Unfortunately, improved contraceptives and easier abortion, to say nothing of meddlesome bureaucracy, have made adoption much more difficult which, even though the world is overpopulated, is sad.

A last word about fertility is that it falls off with age and after thirty in women. As professional people tend to perhaps marry later than some others, it is wise not to wait too long before testing one's fertility, thus allowing time during the persistance of reasonable fertility, for investigation and treatment.

Menopause

Between 45 and 50 the woman's reproductive cycle tends to run down, partly because the ovaries get used up. The periods become irregular and scanty. Various other changes occur including a redistribution of fat to make the figure rounder. All this is called the menopause or change of life. It is totally natural and inevitable and there is no point in resenting it. Unfortunately, the run-down period, which may last for a year or so, can become one of considerable instability. This affects both the emotions and some of the physical systems like vasomotor control. The menopausal woman may be subject to sudden and dramatic 'hot flushes' which are embarrassing and mildly alarming. The emotional instability is shared by the family and many husbands tell me that their wives are trying and irritable, often for far too long.

Any menopausal symptoms that are more than mild or last for more than six months should be treated. Proper hormone replacement therapy, orally and locally if there is post-coital bleeding, should, perhaps with mild tranquillizers, almost completely relieve most of the symptoms. Unfortunately, because most doctors are men and because the change of life tends to become the dumping ground for all the discontents, tensions and disappointments of middle age, treatment of genuine menopausal symptoms tends to be neglected. Otherwise, they need assessing on a psychosomatic basis. It may be essential to find a sympathetic and expert doctor, and they do exist, to deal with the situation.

Contrary to some popular belief, the menopause does not herald the end of sexual enjoyment. Indeed, freed from any fear of pregnancy, it may even be enhanced. As already mentioned, sexual needs vary enormously with age, temperament and previous usage, but certainly they should persist well after the change of life. Women need to know when they can stop taking precautions about becoming pregnant, in relation to the menopause. The usual teaching is that after twelve periods have been missed, it is no longer possible to become pregnant. This is good safe advice, but this is neither an area nor a time of life at which it is sensible to take risks.

Breast cancer

Lastly, we must briefly mention breast cancer. Perhaps because of the continual cyclical changes that the breasts experience, this is the commonest cancer in women. Until recently, the results of treatment were disappointing, largely because this was left too late, often due to the fact that advice was not sought in time because of the fear of cancer.

We now know that if treated early, before it has spread outside the breast, the cure rate can be over 85 per cent. This depends on early detection and we now have the means to do this by regular self-examination, x-ray and what is called thermography or temperature measurement. The next few years will see the rapid development of breast screening centres and the service will hopefully become as available as those for cervical smears and mass chest x-rays. Breast cancer is four times as common as cervical cancer, thus adequate screening is four times as relevant, but still our dilatory ministry of so-called health drags its feet.

Private medicine has established centres in London and Newcastle and the NHS is at last looking at pilot schemes. We have two centres, one in London and one mobile, and perhaps we shall have the resources to expand these. Like the reduction of IHD, for me, this is the most exciting growth area in preventive medicine and it is hoped that women will themselves demand the extension of the facilities.

To achieve this, women must themselves learn to live with the possibility that they might develop the condition. They must literally learn their way round their breasts and by regular, every month, self-examination, pick up the minute changes that may herald a treatable cancer. Cancer is no longer a death sentence, nor does it necessarily mean a disfiguring operation. For reasons already given, breasts can become tender, lumpy and nodular. Not all small lumps are malignant, but all discrete palpable lumps and other tender areas may harbour a cancer. The only way to be sure about what they are is literally to have them out and look at them under a microscope. If this toll is to be reduced, and surely it can be, women must firstly learn systematic self-examination, secondly, attend a screening centre about once a year after the age of forty and, thirdly, accept the possibility of a small biopsy operation, should a lump be found, without getting into a frenzy of anxiety about dying of cancer. To detect over fifty early cancers in about 7000 women, we advised just over three times this number of biopsies. By doing this we hope that we have not only saved these fifty or so women a lot of turmoil and possible death, but we have also indoctrinated the whole 7000 into self-examination. American experience shows that when indoctrinated in this way, the women themselves become the best detectors of their own early cancers, because they cannot be x-rayed monthly, even in an ideal state.

Woman's role in the future

For reasons we do not understand, women may be tougher than men, but they do have a number of particular medical problem areas which demand more understanding and better treatment than they often get.

Women have fewer medical hazards than men and have the edge over them for longevity, as can be seen from Figures 1:1 and 1:3. With wider education, freedom to travel, improved contraception and a lessening of social pressure to find their only role in home and family, it will be interesting to see what the next fifty years bring to women's lot. Certainly women need to bring to bear on society the benefits of their improved position if we are not to inhabit a world 'top-heavy' with chronically sick, elderly females, a sight that is already too familiar in our hospitals, nursing homes and sheltered housing establishments.

In short, women must not mistake equality for quality. We in preventive medicine believe that quality and quantity go hand in hand, both for men and women.

THIRTEEN

Living Sensibly

Attitudes to and disciplines of working

One of my most worn-out looking patients was an unfortunate who was running a small UK subsidiary of an unperceptive and uncongenial American conglomerate (although it was not called that in those days). This man said that he spent Mondays through to Fridays keeping the Americans quiet and ran the company Saturdays and Sundays, which was no way of life, particularly with quarterly visits to 'Big Brother' in New York. In this latter respect, he soon found it wise to travel Friday night and hole up in New York until Monday morning: otherwise he was beaten before he started.

Clearly, this was no way to live and he had the good sense to get into a less demanding and more congenial job. Otherwise, he was very much at hazard. But we do see people periodically who have to be 'dug out' of work situations which are too taxing. Sometimes, however, we are too late and it is the coronary or nervous breakdown that produces the crisis.

The trouble with work patterns is that they are taken for granted and allowed to grow, or evolve, like Topsy. An ill thought out and poorly organized work pattern that gets by, up to early middle age, may well become critical as the man gets older. The shrewd executive and sensible senior manager should see that he personally, and his youngsters on the way up, learn to work effectively and within a margin, so that they have something in reserve for a crisis.

Because so little thought or training is given to methods of and attitudes towards work in general, I am going to stick my medical neck out and discuss some of the areas that seem to me to cause stress and difficulty.

Learning how to work

Someone who has had a professional or academic training, be this an arts degree, an articled apprenticeship in, say, accountancy, or a sandwich course in engineering, starts with a number of advantages. The biggest of these is that he has been given a discipline or framework within which to organize both his time and his methods of actually doing the job. The other great benefit that a professional training should bestow is the tradition of being able to find out what you do not know; thus consulting reference works, keeping up to date, going to lectures and courses, etc, becomes a familiar habit. Without this habit, there is a tendency to protect ignorance by a reluctance to expose it.

This ability is becoming increasingly important and it is being realized now that in all walks of life, in order to live with today's rate of change, we need the understanding of 'learning to learn throughout life'. It is being said that individuals should be flexible enough to do three jobs in their life times. This should include the final perception to go into retirement with enough skills and activities to preserve sanity. An additional advantage of this philosophy is that it makes the acceptance of technological change more acceptable. Over the last decade, many managers have been seriously stressed by their fear of computers and the bright young men that allegedly understand them.

Most of this comes easily to the 'professional' and will become easier for the better trained manager of tomorrow. But todays management is still, to a large extent, made up of self-made men who have come up the hard way. Many of them left school relatively early and have done outstandingly well with limited educational resources. As time goes on and the demands of their work becomes more administrative and institutional and less entrepreneurial, their lack of the right skills can be very stressful.

I believe that organizations should now give much more thought to the simple systems and traditions under which their younger staff develop. Somehow or other, people are expected to know how to dictate a letter, work a filing system, write decent English, understand a balance sheet and compose a cogent report. That in practice rather few people can do any of these things well is apparent in the output and method of functioning of most organizations.

It seems extremely likely that there would be less stress in later life, and perhaps fewer failures in communication all round, if better working disciplines were insisted on for the younger staff in all organizations. These would then be carried forward to make the later half of life easier and would hopefully be copied more or less as automatically as bad habits now are. This may become even more necessary with sloppier educational standards and the unwillingness of the young to accept the educational disciplines of 'the three Rs'. Even university graduates now often get degrees without being seemingly able to write simple English.

It is suggested that this area is looked at under the following headings and against the general background of learning to learn and keeping up to date.

The written word

Largely fortuitously, I spent the war doing what was then called operational research. As part of my training, I learnt to write reports which were made to have a beginning, middle and end. This skill has stood me in good stead ever since, and I still get worried by my doctors and other colleagues who produce waffly and high sounding but meaningless reports and letters. The value of this was brought home to me early in my Institute of Directors life when we dealt with proportionately more self-made men who were brave enough to admit that their inability to express themselves in words was becoming a limiting factor in their growth. It is quite a revealing exercise for instance to take the secretaries out for a drink and discover how few of the people they work for are competent 'dictators and writers'. It is a waste of expensive secretarial time to have draft after draft retyped because the originator neither knows what he wants to say or is able to say it.

It seems imperative that knowledge along these lines should be made part of the tradition of working: that commercial jargon should be penalized and all incoming mail at least acknowledged, if not answered, within 48 hours.

Social skills and speaking

Those of us who arrived at the age of, say 25, able to go as a stranger to a cocktail party, make a short speech or chair a simple meeting, have no idea how lucky we are. We were able, through our early backgrounds to absorb these skills without really noticing. An able businessman, who has done well for himself, but came from a working-class background, will tell you how difficult it is to behave comfortably in these circumstances.

Over the years, looking for sources of stress in people who are up against various margins, this has often been found to be a limiting factor of which they were rather ashamed. One very able man, who was technically a leader in his field, had refused appointment to a 'little Neddy' because he and his wife were too stressed by the social and other demands of life in this new league.

It seems that a great deal still needs to be done to bridge some of the differences in behaviour which our growing social mobility has produced. This can be particularly true for wives. The self-made man, tends, or some of them do, to marry early and from his own background. He is lucky indeed if his wife has the same growth potential as he has. Mostly they do not and this can produce a very traumatic conflict in loyalties.

Planning the day: having priorities

One of the bugbears of modern business life is the concept of the 'open door'. That people are encouraged to drop in, means that the 'boss' is not allowed to get on with anything consistently unless he is actually at a meeting. Incidentally, how many of these are really necessary?

If he is to survive at the top, it is essential for an executive to acquire a tidy mind and good working disciplines. This involves setting a series of priorities, getting on with the jobs systematically, minimizing personal and telephone interruptions and being organized by a good secretary. 'The dragon in the outer office' and having all phone calls filtered are extremely helpful.

Part of this process, and very much part of my executive administration kit, is the delegation drill. The willingness to delegate comes easily only to the secure and perhaps the lazy. But part of growing old gracefully is to push the work down the line while keeping the strings in your hands. Self-made people and promoted 'doers', rather than organizers, find this a very difficult skill to acquire. The successful line manager who becomes an administrator finds it very difficult to adjust to not having anything to actually operate. Unless he can learn fairly quickly he will destroy both himself and those under him by interfering.

I am personally very sensitive to working environment and am prepared to take trouble and if necessary to spend a little of my own money on making my office a pleasant place. When we started The Medical Centre I bought a splendid picture which I took to the office rather than leave at home, as I suddenly realized that we all spend more of our waking lives in the office than we do at home.

More thought should be given to making offices peaceful and pleasant, especially now that rents are so high. In visiting an organization for the first time, I always make a point of looking at it critically, starting at reception and going right through to the man in his office. To what extent does this express his personality and method of working? It is interesting how often, presumably because she cares, the secretary's office is nicer than that of the boss. Many of our senior offices are bleak and impersonal. It seems that Americans tend to be better at this than we are, perhaps because they are more concerned about status symbols.

There appears to be a tendency for executives in relation to themselves and the way in which they let those below them operate, to pay too little attention to how they actually spend their time. It is disastrously easy to get sucked into spending far too much energy on trivial but satisfying routine, at the expense of the difficult things and forward planning. We would all benefit from more 'think time' in which to get things into better perspective. My ideal state would include almost a day a week spent working peacefully at home rather than in the office. It is surprising how much can be done in this way. Much more 'think time' would be a major stress reducer. It would be achieved by the ruthless pruning of unnecessary meetings, better management of essential ones and the elimination of purely bureaucratic paper. All sadly and probably unachievably utopian.

What counts as work

Clinically, in making our environmental assessment we divide life into work, home and leisure. If Mr. Average is asked, 'What do you do when you are not working?', the answering look is mostly blank. The need for and value of relaxational pursuits is discussed elsewhere, but it is difficult for the professional man to draw a line between work and social activities.

When I was more of a practising doctor, I used to be a regular attender at medical meetings, partly to represent the organization for which I worked and partly hopefully to improve my mind. Soon one gets sucked into the organization of these meetings and the running of professional groups. All this is legitimately regarded as work and to a degree should be encouraged. Companies are, on the whole, good about letting senior people participate in this way and presumably it is good for the image of the company. There may be a similar case for more public and community participation, in company time.

Going to meetings, reading journals and keeping up to date is certainly work but what about entertaining and being entertained? This is certainly work too and needs strictly controlling. A sensible rule is that no man should be out more than two nights a week. If he is, he should take his wife with him at least once. As a man gets older he should devote more time to local and community things and less to those more directly business and professional. His basic skills can be immensely helpful in this area; it is good for him to play a perhaps less dominant role and again he must build up contacts and activities which are not specifically work related.

If most of what we do counts as work, it is obviously desirable to see that we do not do too much of it. There are plenty of examples of rather pathetic but well-known tycoons who are so badly organized and so unable to delegate that they get to the office at 7 am and leave in time for a late supper. This degree of involvement cannot really be necessary and it is unlikely that this type of man will make old bones. Senior people are employed to take decisions and give advice. The good ones have empty desks, are easy to get hold of and devote a proportion of their energies to government and other committees.

An undesirable feature of the insecure man is 'the first in last out complex'. He must demonstrate how much harder he works than anyone else and how indispensable he is. Unless he really is a one-man band, he is pathetic rather than meritorious. Long hours may be necessary for some people sometimes, but not really for those at the top. There are three reasons for staying late, to avoid the traffic, to get things done peacefully without the phone going and to save taking work home. Probably time is in fact wasted during the day, but the pattern is only acceptable if it is associated with a late start.

Eating, drinking and smoking

Preventive medicine hinges largely round health education which, in its turn, is a problem of communication and motivation similar to marketing and public relations exercises. The problem is, as always, how does one motivate people to change their way of life and give up some of the pleasures of over-indulgence?

Over the years, The Medical Centre has been modestly successful in dealing with at least two of these problems (reliable figures on alcohol consumption are virtually impossible to obtain) in two ways. First, by helping to create a general climate of opinion based on a greater realization of the problems involved. And then within this climate, to motivate individuals to set an example and optimize their own health. Over the years, we have used the sort of statistics quoted in Part One which do illustrate the hazards and disadvantages of 'the sin'. Businessmen are used to making quality judgements on the basis of facts and figures and this has been a help. In addition, we have rather fierce booklets on weight, smoking, cholesterol and exercise, and we recommend that each person takes these home to discuss them with his wife.

Over the years, about a quarter of the cigarette smokers we see (who are about half the total attenders) are persuaded to stop or cut for periods of over a year (the minimum to qualify for the statistics) and more than a third of the overweights manage to reduce. The figures for smoking are shown in Figure 2:12.

It is legitimate to use group solidarity and company traditions to deal with some of the potential excesses of smoking, drinking and over-eating. Senior people, from the chaiman downwards, can and should set examples and standards and, if necessary, register a certain amount of disapproval. This is not interfering with individual liberties, it is the prudence of protecting the company's assets.

It is, for instance, well known that certain firms tend to be over-indulgent in the directors' or executive dining room, or to drink large quantities of gin after six o'clock. This nearly always stems from one or two people who really ought to know better. And it is often very difficult for the younger executives not to swim along with the tide.

Weight

For most people, weight control is very much a question of calorie book-keeping. If you consume more calories than you need, they are banked away as fat. Different builds or types of people use their calories slightly differently. The thin, rather manic types burn up their energy because they tick over at a higher rate. Most of the rest of us are just good converters and have to be careful over our book-keeping.

Eating is undoubtedly a major pleasure and one which persists throughout life. Equally eating is very much a series of habits. We get used to eating certain quantities of certain foods, at given times, and then miss their absence. Thus both hunger and desire for food is based on habit reflexes. It is easy, by various refined gimmicks in starvation, to get people to lose weight quite dramatically. (Dietetically there is little difference between health farms and concentration camps, except the orange juice and bowel washouts.) But once they return to their previous way of life, back goes the weight. They bounce up and down like a yo-yo.

In fact, weight can only be kept under control by a discipline which gets the weight down gradually over several months and at the same time redeploys eating habits to keep it at a reasonable level. Once the new habit pattern is established, it becomes little hardship. Obviously, it is better if the whole family joins the new regime.

Interestingly, in the last ten years or so, it has been learnt that fat babies make fat children, fat children obese adults. In addition, the eating habits that parents inflict on their children get transferred to the next adult generation. Thus, sensible attitudes to children's diets are very important and the use of carbohydrate-rich convenience foods, as particularly in America, must be discouraged. It is known also that overweight children and adults tend to be physically inactive.

Another interesting trend emerging in our society at the moment is that the members of the professional classes are more health conscious than those in social classes IV and V. There is a growing volume of evidence which suggests that the proportion of obesity in these classes of people is much higher. Chips with everything, rigidity about certain foods, coupled with a disinclination to try anything different, makes for obesity.

Calorie book-keeping should be done over the week and not on a day-to-day basis. This gives much more flexibility and allows for the occasional pleasure of the over-indulgent blow-out. Businessmen and others who have to do a lot of wining and dining (most of them need not really do as much as their image of themselves presupposes) must compensate by eating less at the weekends. Thus a heavy week at the office must be compensated by an ambstemious weekend.

In achieving a sensible weekly calorie balance the cooperation and understanding of the wife is essential. Here considerable conflict can arise because, to a degree, almost the only way in which a wife can display her skill and maintain her job satisfaction is by producing rather splendid meals; a situation often made worse by the fact that this could be her main meal. But on the whole tired middle-aged businessmen prefer and do better on light suppers.

Breakfast is a very important meal. Although the human animal is so adaptable that it can be trained for almost anything, like living on grass and apples, or one meal a day, it is basically designed to take on fuel at regular intervals. As it is a very long time from dinner at night to lunch the next day, breakfast does help to balance things out. Lunch seems to be the best meal to cut down on, but this is not always possible. And it is important to have a break in the middle of the day.

The main source of energy in the body comes from sugar in the blood. The level goes up after meals and drops quite low with hunger. Low levels also contribute to feeling limp, tired and sometimes a bit remote. Thin people, for instance, who sometimes tend to eat too little, get very low at the end of the day. Having a few sweets in the car to eat on the way home, often helps here, and they can afford this indulgence.

Thus, the first key to weight control is a balanced meal pattern. If weight control is a problem, as it is for most of people, within this pattern, bread, potatoes, sugar and puddings must be reduced. Weight control is very much a matter of looking after the calorie pennies and leaving the pounds to care for themselves.

A good starting point is to cut out sugar in tea and coffee. One tea addict regularly had over 20 lumps of sugar a day in the tea supplied by doting wife and secretary. One very soon gets used to sweeteners like Saxin. If, for example bread and potatoes are no problem but you adore puddings, then allow yourself two or so a week. The trick is to perm the allowable, by eating the things you like and enjoy, and cutting out the others. Fried foods are more fattening than grilled, and lean meat than fat meat. Remember too, that alcohol is a high calorie food, so if it is chosen something else has to go.

Diets are ten a penny and most of them perm calories in a variety of ways. In the end they can only work by reducing the total calorie intake. How this is done matters rather little.

Not only is eating a major pleasure, it is also a source of comfort. Many seriously overweight people are compulsive eaters, because they are inherently insecure. Others go on an 'eating blind' when they get unhappy or have a crisis. Very seriously overweight people pose considerable medical and psychological problems and are in practice very difficult to cure or help. They are taken into hospital for several months and their weights reduced from, say, eighteen to eleven stone, but the moment they get home it all goes back on again. We have had one or two outstanding successes with

Weight-watchers. This organization combines a sensible dietary regime with the group solidarity of the public confessional. On the whole, it is more acceptable to women than to men, but men can and do use it successfully.

For most of people, there are two golden rules about weight control. The first is to know roughly what your weight should be and to understand the reasons for keeping it down. Insurance companies issue 'height, weight, age tables' and some of these are further adjusted for body and bone structure. But these tables are based on average weight for groups of people; in fact, most of them come from the American Life Insurance Companies because sadly their English counterparts are not interested enough to produce any medically useful figures. But the optimum weight for 'you' is best judged by a doctor working along the lines outlined in Chapter 3. This gives you an aiming mark. The next step is to be sure to have a reasonably accurate pair of bathroom scales. Weigh yourself weekly at roughly the same time of day. Once you have got down to 'bogey', the absolute weight matters less than keeping it stable. Even fairly inaccurate scales are good enough for the weekly pound or two. But do not let it creep slowly up, just because it is too cold to play golf or cut the lawn.

The second rule is to get your eating pattern organized so as to keep your weight in balance without too much hardship. This will require the cooperation of your wife and self-discipline on your part. No nibbling between meals, no second helpings and no bread or potatoes. One of the benefits about eating out a lot is that it is fairly easy to pick and choose expensive low-calorie menus. Melon, steak, cold meat and salad, grilled fish, fruit and cheese are all perfectly acceptable.

Appetite suppressant pills and sometimes mild sedatives do have a modest role in helping the early stages of weight control. They are a prop, but no substitute for resolve, and in the end it is resolve that will win the day.

Quite a lot of people make regular visits to health farms. These come in various shapes, sizes and price ranges. The gimmicks apart, they all work on the basis of selling starvation. Mostly they are so relatively expensive that no-one will admit to having wasted their money. Seriously, fat people can lose nearly a stone in a fortnight, but so they could at home. As already mentioned, the real trouble with these places is that although you get weight down, it soon comes back again because it is not a new way of life.

Health farms and hydros may be an expensive way of losing weight, but they do have a role for the obsessive type of person who will not take a holiday but would accept a medically-oriented break. Although he may be the man who sneaks out for the beer and steak that is available within a mile of all these places, it is better that he should go there than stay in the office. By a strange quirk of behaviour, this man will accept the slightly odd discipline of the hydro, whereas no-one at home, or at work, can conceivably tell *him* what to do.

One last point, remember that all you lose in a Turkish or Sauna bath is sweat, and this loss is soon replaced by drinking.

Alcohol

I am strongly in favour of alcohol in reasonable quantities. It is a tranquillizer, a social lubricant and a pleasure to consume. But it is a drug of addiction, a high-calorie food and potential social disruptant. There is also no doubt that although it loosens up inhibitions and shyness, in more than limited amounts it undoubtedly diminishes performance.

Ten years ago the heavy business lunch was a legitimate cartoon target. Although it is still desirable to make semi-social contact the amount of food and drink consumed has diminished considerably. Businessmen are not idle and the real problem is that the long lunch tends to lengthen the day.

Practically all of us are socially competent drinkers and we know, and practically never exceed, the amount we can take on a given occasion, ie one can drink more at home on New Year's Eve than at a city dinner. But there are a few people who slip down the slope and become alcohol dependent or overt alcoholics. After 15-20 years, the vulnerable and weaker ones get into the habit of being partially anaesthetized, so that drinking becomes both a prop and a poison. But there is no doubt that the rest of us, without becoming alcoholics can, unless we are careful, easily get into something of the same habit pattern and begin to drink more than we need or is good for us.

Without becoming either paranoid or 'precious' about it, it must always be remembered that alcohol is an insidious mistress and, if one is in the sort of work/social situation where drink tends to happen at lunch and in the evening, to be very careful about how much one has and how often. It is also reassuring to prove to oneself that it is possible to go without, at least over the odd weekend or for several days at a time. I used to have lunch with a senior advertising man at a restaurant where he was well known. The waiter used to say 'Your usual Mr . . .' and it took me a long time to discover that his 'usual' was a tonic without gin.

It is also worth remembering that it takes many years of moderate drinking to make an alcoholic; alcoholics are made as much as born, which is why senior individuals and organizations do have a responsibility to set sensible standards and to actively discourage over-indulgence.

Industry is currently being blamed for some of the alcoholism that is said to be prevalent. In as much as it employs alcoholics, it is obviously involved in the situation. And there is no doubt that the occasional alcoholic is found at various levels in a number of firms. I think that as employers we have two responsibilities, firstly to discourage too much drinking and, secondly, to deal, much more firmly with those whose performance is diminished by over-indulgence.

At The Medical Centre, we run a very sophisticated quality-control procedure on the various tests that we do, and a couple of years ago we were fascinated to find that the mean level of one of the liver function tests was well above normal, on January 1st. This meant three things: first, that our control mechanism was sensitive; second, so was the test for liver damage by alcohol and third, that the mean level of liver damage on New Year's Eve had been too high. In practice, we do find that a number of regular heavy drinkers are giving their livers a heavier burden than they can carry. Usually, showing them the figures from their tests is all that is required to discourage them from drinking so much.

There are one or two useful points about drinking that are worth mentioning. The physiological or disinhibiting effect of alcohol on the brain comes from the actual chemical, ethyl alcohol (C_2H_5OH). What goes with it, in terms of taste, etc, is hooked on chemically, but has little to do with the chemical effect.

Alcohol is rapidly absorbed from an empty stomach, which at the time has nothing else to do, and much less rapidly when competing with food, particularly fatty food, for absorption. It is also said that mashed potato is good blotting paper because it holds the drink like a sponge. Strong alcohol is obviously more irritant to the stomach than dilute and in addition requires to be diluted by body fluid. Like coffee, alcohol is also a diaretic, ie it stimulates the kidneys to get rid of it, which also requires fluid. Thus, it is better to take diluted rather than concentrated drink and it is very wise after a heavy night to take a good drink of water before going to bed.

Hangovers are multifactorial, but the two main features are dehydration and stomach or gastric irritation. The vomiting and the queasiness are due to the direct irritant effect on the stomach. Plenty of water and alkali such as Alka Seltzer helps here. The main reason why a true alcoholic gets cirrhosis may be because he gets deficiency diseases of vitamins and protein. Because his stomach is constantly inflamed, he not only feels awful, but cannot bring himself to eat. A vicious circle is set up under which, because of the gastritis, he does not feel human until he has had a drink, which leads to another drink, which means that he tends not to have a proper meal and lives on 'pub snacks'.

Alcohol is absorbed and distributed throughout the body. Some is lost in the breath and urine, hence the medico-legal tests. But the main reservoir is held in the blood and detoxicated by the liver. Clearly as the liver gets damaged or over-worked, detoxication takes longer and so alcohol levels remain raised and the individual remains fuddled. The probability is that blood levels in established alcoholics never get back low enough to allow them legally to drive a car. Similarly, many people, after a very heavy night, ought not to drive to work in the mornings. Luckily, the breathalysers are seldom out at that hour. The process of digestion, also speeds up the oxydation and disposal of alcohol. Thus a meal has a double benefit; delayed absorption and more rapid removal.

Alcohol is a vasodilator, ie it opens the blood vessels, particularly those in the skin. This is why one gets a bit red in the face after a couple of drinks and also may sweat. Thus, on the whole, alcohol is good or at least does no harm for arteriosclerosis and coronary ischaemia. It should not be given to shocked or cold people unless they are in the warm, because it diverts blood to the skin and puts up heat loss, the feeling or warmth being illusory.

Apart from the wisdom of diluting alcohol and avoiding American-type cocktails, it must be realized that many of the calories come from what goes with the drink. Sweet drinks are more fattening than dry drinks and squash or bitter lemon has more calories than soda water or tonic. It is also wise in terms of counting the calorie pennies, to have slimline or low-calorie soft drinks and, if there is a real problem diabetic squash. For most of us, however, modest quantities of alcohol may better than bread and potatoes.

Alcoholism is commoner on the Continent than it is in England. There seem to be two reasons for this: cost and way of life. The French, for instance, are brought up on alcohol and its addictiveness does the rest, without there being an appreciable number of drunks about the place. These factors, however, do not apply in Scandinavia and America, where alcoholism is commoner than it is in England. Undoubtedly the general sense of insecurity and rat-race life in the USA contributes to this and American industry is so worried about the problem that many firms forbid all drink on the premises, and have anti-drug and anti-alcohol programmes run by their medical departments.

Alcohol can be a dangerous mistress and it is wise to be on personal guard against sliding into heavy drinking habits. It is also desirable, on the one hand, to set sensible standards within the organization and, on the other, to deal very firmly with the known malefactor. Somebody, and it can only be the organization, owes it to him to protect him from disgrace and self destruction.

Smoking

Little more need be said about smoking cigarettes. They are positively lethal, but obviously satisfying. There is little evidence that the intense anti-smoking propaganda is having any overall effect on reducing national cigarette consumption. It is clearly almost impossible to frighten cigarette addicts into stopping. Our experience is that the much more real risk of coronary thrombosis is a better motivator than the much smaller risk of lung cancer. It is particularly important to try to stop children smoking up to the age of 18.

There are few substitutes for resolve in stopping smoking. The various pills available are probably no use, except possibly as a short term prop. Tranquillizers may help too in the short term. Hypnotism very seldom helps, and all the other many and various cures have their supporters, but they merely provide the framework on which to hang resolve.

Sometimes one can trigger this off by saying, 'Mr. Y. I bet you will not leave your cigarettes with the receptionist and never have another'. At other times, illness, cough, cardiograph change or a coronary in firm or family will trigger off stopping.

The probability is, and there are always exceptions, that because of its addictiveness, it is unwise and impossible just to cut down; one must be brave and stop altogether. For similar reasons, very few cigarette smokers manage to transfer to pipe or cigars. The temptation is still too close and inhaling these two is possibly more dangerous even than cigarettes, because the smoke is more irritant. A recent case was that of a man with a noisy chest, who inhaled 15 cigars a day.

As far as we know, pipes and cigars, not inhaled and taken in reasonable quantity, are safe, as are 1-3 cigarettes a day, provided the number does not creep up.

Two last points concern the problems of stopping smoking and the prohibiting of smoking. Firstly, as it is an addiction, it is likely that sudden stopping will produce the same medical symptoms as will the sudden withdrawal of any other drug of addiction, known as acute withdrawal symptoms. Indeed it does, and very alarming they can be. The cigarette smoker who stops must expect and so must his family, a fairly miserable fortnight. He will be irritable, bloody minded, paranoid, depressed, etc, and all his worst faults will be magnified. Concentration and sleep may be interfered with. It is thus often difficult to attempt stopping at a difficult time when at work. Perhaps, hell though it may be for the family, a holiday is the best time to start the cure.

A recent patient went off to a health farm to stop smoking. I knew that he drank a fair amount but did not realize quite how much. The sudden withdrawal of both drugs, produced an acute psychiatric situation, which had to be separately and urgently dealt with. Another patient, an artist, smoked 50 cigarettes a day. He requested a hypnotist, but two days later his wife rang up to say that he had been curled up on the couch in his studio looking at the wall. The treatment was, and can be, worse than the disease. We had to dehypnotize him.

Secondly to what extent should individuals, organizations and institutions make it more difficult to smoke? Mr Heath apparently did not allow smoking at cabinet meetings: should we allow them at business and board meetings, in offices and public places? It is also worth remembering that smoking at work is a post-war phenomenon; before then one went to the lavatory for a drag. Should we get back to this?

Exercise

The main reasons for taking an adequate amount of exercise regularly are as follows:

1   It develops a cardiac reserve and, to a degree, protects against coronary thrombosis. Sedentary people have a higher IHD rate than those who are physically active.
2   It keeps bones and joints supple and mobile.
3   It maintains and develops muscle strength.
4   The resulting physical fitness and discipline required to maintain it, have an additional moral value in that fit people feel better, are better for a variety of medical reasons and almost certainly perform better.

A fifth point which might be added is that it is far more difficult for fat people to get fit than it is for thin ones. Thus, exercise is an aid to weight control and it does use up a few calories.

Another good reason, particularly after the age of 55, is that if one wants to remain spry and active into retirement, it is necessary to *get* active well before retirement. Fitness 'in hand' can be retained but fitness lost is hard to retrieve.

There are always exceptions to all rules and people do survive without much exercise, but many more are better for taking it. Really it is never too late to start. If you puff too easily, or get chest pain or ache and creak after the slightest activity, see a doctor before you start getting fit. In most large centres now, there are gymnasia where qualified instructors can turn the flabbiest middle-aged mortal into a better going concern. They usually have classes for men in this condition and do not expect them to compete with the young, or the keep-fit ladies. Modern gymnasia, not the sauna massage traps, tend not to smell of feet and have various enjoyable gadgetry to make all the bits of you work.

But gymnasia apart, two things are required for the exercise regime. The first is that there should be a bend and stretch element to put all the joints through their full range of movement. The second is general physical activity to 'use' the muscles, build up their strength and make the heart work.

A number of PT regimes have been well written up. Probably the best is the Canadian 5BX regime available as a Penguin book. This schedule is infinitely boring, takes about 12 minutes a day and should be done 4-5 times a week, but it does work.

Exercise machines, static bicycles, rowing machines, etc, are all acceptable, so is brisk walking, swimming, gardening, golf and other games. In fact, anything that gets you out into the open and is enjoyed is acceptable. Half an hour a day is to be aimed at. Dogs help because they have to be exercised, but a slow lamp-post crawl with a snuffling peke is not much good.

Older people who do regular physical work (such as gardeners) retain prodigious strength late into life. I have several patients over 70, who play gentle family tennis, and one of them has had a coronary. Usually golf is reasonable exercise, but it can become an over-social extension of the office work group, and calorie consuming at the bar afterwards.

Obviously, exercise tends to be concentrated at the weekends, but some walking during the week is highly desirable, particularly if one is away from home. Americans who never walk anywhere, are always surprised when one arrives or leaves on foot.

Being reasonably active is also an attitude of mind; walk part of the way to work, do not use the lift, go and see people, charge about the place a bit. It all helps and others might emulate you. Stair climbing can be used as a good guide to fitness. Count the level at which you puff and measure the improvement a month later.

Although it sounds simple and trivial, one of my most rewarding pieces of preventive medicine was to persuade a 50-year-old man to lose 1½ stones, stop smoking and take regular exercise. He moved to Richmond, bought a dog and took it out in the park twice a day. In three months he became a new, better and much more effective man. Liveliness of body must to a degree, be reflected in liveliness of mind.

Commuting

I have a bee in my bonnet about commuting. I know that it is a London disease and living on the fringes is cheaper and less unpleasant. But two hours a day spent in travel is ten hours a week, which is a lot of working time and energy. Three hours a day, not all that uncommon, is two working days wasted on travel, and the reading can be done elsewhere, in less unpleasant surroundings.

Obviously, family needs and preferences, schools, etc, all come into this. But difficult though it is, at around 55, the energy and anxiety squandered on commuting should be seriously considered. The London flat, even for two or three nights a week, or the house on a direct tubeline is also a help.

Driving in and out of London is becoming increasingly demanding. Anyone of reasonable seniority who drives himself much more than ten thousand miles a year for work needs his priorities looked at. What is he employed for and how should his time and energy be spent? A recent example was that of a very worn-out company chairman, who habitually drove himself from Dundee to Glasgow for meetings. With a chauffer he could work one way and sleep the other and be far less tired at the end of the week.

One man was persuaded to move into London when the children grew up. They got a London flat, went out in the evenings and his wife went back to the Stockbroker belt for her social activities and commitments. As she travelled against the tide, it was easy. It completely changed the energy they both have available to spend on enjoyment.

Holidays

Industry and commerce, compared with the universities, public service, etc, are thoroughly mean about holidays, and Americans and Continentals are even worse.

When we did our original Institute of Directors survey in 1959, around a third of these replying had two weeks or less, which is less than they had to give to keep a London secretary. Things have now improved somewhat and 3-4 weeks is average. Senior people with a lot of responsibility really should have 4-6 weeks. They need the break to think things out and it is very good for the staff to get on without them.

Because people's inclinations and requirements vary, generalization about holidays is dangerous. A few people, particularly self-made men, get bored after much more than a long weekend; they literally do not know what to do with themselves. The sole relaxation of one distinguished surgeon was to take the night sleeper to Aberdeen, walk on the moors all day and then sleeper back. Some people take a week to unwind and relax, others switch off the moment they get away. Money and children come into it too, but as a general rule, at least two holidays a year is advocated, one long and one shorter. Long weekends, with days tacked on to Christmas and Easter and, if at all possible, staff at all levels should be encouraged to take odd days off as well. If they cannot be trusted to work hard, they may well not be worth employing. Again, as one gets older, it is false economy to work 49 weeks and rest for three. The year requires to be divided up into more equal slices and an early spring holiday is a marvellous relief after the English winter.

Couples with children need 'one spade and bucket' expedition and one break for parents without the children. Older people might well benefit (perish the thought) from a break without each other. Men who travel can tack breaks on to the end of trips and have their wives join them. Men who travel a lot should have a trip a year with their wives and stop somewhere nice.

Academic life assumes that people who use their brains, and some of them do, benefit from a break away from the grindstone. This is called sabbatical leave and, strictly speaking, should happen every seven years. A few enlightened firms do give some of their people a break to recharge their batteries and this seems to be a very desirable practice. Such leave is not an extra holiday; it is a chance to get away from the daily rat race and do something different, see how the other half live and collect new ideas and perspectives. It requires an act of imagination from a bureaucrat to create the precedent of paying someone for three months for doing nothing of obvious benefit, but there could be enormous advantages. It seems quite certain that the practice will spread and, hopefully, a greater number of managers will be equipped to know what to do with themselves.

Activities outside work

The importance for the middle aged of involvement in activities and interests outside their work has already been mentioned and emphasized. It is only mentioned again here because it is a vital part of living sensibly. The work-centred man is boring and vulnerable, we suspect he dies young and we know he is unhappy when he retires. In my view, everyone over the age of 50 should have extra curricular involvements which will carry over into retirement. Businessmen, who misunderstand and are misunderstood by the community, tend to be accused of being only interested in making money. This may be true of a few of them, but the concept of ploughing something back into the community and using their skills to improve the quality of life for others, is one which is well worth encouraging.

In addition, it is very good for the tycoon at work to be a humbler part of, say, the Parish Council or a local Abbeyfield Society. And he should be encouraged to really participate and not just write a cheque. In point of fact, many of these people, if they can be got away from their own work, have very usable talents and skills. One of the troubles is that they are used to dominating and do not tolerate the 'fool on the committee' gladly, but it is good for them to try. Even winning a prize at the local rose show is good for morale. A famous French surgeon who had a country house in a non-vintage wine area also grew his own wine, which was very good. He took a malicious pleasure in taking it up to Paris in unlabelled bottles, transferring it to a decanter, and trying some on his smart friends.

People who have brains should use them in more than one sphere.

One other vital area of living sensibly is health maintenance examinations, considered in the next chapter.

FOURTEEN
Health Maintenance Examinations

Declaring, in the best parliamentary tradition, my interest in 'the health check', one can now claim that preventive maintenance on people is a sensible and justifiable procedure. Most of us visit the dentist regularly, and without necessarily waiting for something to go obviously wrong. Equally, we have our cars serviced regularly, and if the garage recommends replacing something before it breaks, we foot the bill reasonably cheerfully, so that breakdowns on the motorway are hopefully less likely. For the same reasons mechanical devices are subject to regular supervision and preventive maintenance.

The analogy between the car and the human can usefully be pushed a little further. There is no doubt that a car that is persistently driven flat out over longish distances wears out appreciably sooner than one that is not made to function continuously at its maximum capacity. For the same reasons, the mileage that has been covered is some reflection of the 'safe' mileage that is left. So to a degree, it is with people. If a man looks really older than he is (not just a bit grey which might be a family trait), it probably means that he is burning himself out and consequently has little reserve for the future.

As we have said, the young can safely work very hard for ten or fifteen years, but after this it is wise to begin slowing down if one wants to have steam left in the boiler after, say, 55. The health check, by picking up the early mental and physical signs of wear, may sound a warning which, if heeded, can be used to restore some of the lost energy. Unlike worn out machinery, the human animal does have considerable powers of recovery and replacement. Joints worn out with arthritis do not stop creaking, but other changes are increasingly reversible and even joints, heart valves and some of the arteries can now be replaced by grafts or artificial prostheses.

Many of the changes we have discussed in relation to IHD come on insidiously and cause no overt symptoms. It is only by checking the systems like weight, blood pressure, cardiograph, chest x-ray, blood chemistry, etc, that one can detect and quantify early changes. We call this pre-symptomatic diagnosis and it is the cornerstone of preventive medicine. After all, even if one knows what one's weight is and should be, it is only by actually measuring other important indices like cholesterol, that we can know whether they are normal or not.

There is also the possibility of finding other conditions causing symptoms which are being neglected for a variety of reasons. Some of these like varicose veins, haemorrhoids, the need for vision and hearing testing and so on, may not be serious in themselves, but they do detract from general efficiency and benefit from treatment. There is also the long-standing or chronic condition, the dyspepsia, the diabetes, the psoriasis or eczema which have become part of the individual's life. These tend to be accepted by his doctor as being 'chronic stable' and require no new treatment. All these conditions should be looked at and reassessed regularly. The health check provides an opportunity for doing this. Also, long experience has taught me the dangers of a person being labelled with a certain disease, like diabetes. This tends to stop the doctor looking for other conditions. The diabetic is just as much in need of a general service as anyone else, perhaps more so.

The benefits of regular health maintenance, and the arguments in favour of it, can be looked at under three main headings:

1   To the individual and his family
2   To the company
3   To the community as a whole

Because this is so important it is worth looking at these three areas in a little more detail.

Benefit to the individual

We have already looked at, in outline, the arguments in favour of preventive maintenance on people and the vital part that presymptomatic diagnosis plays in making preventive medicine effective and practical. Coronary risk factors are a classical example in men; the forum of the examination can help a person to come to terms with his problems, change his attitudes and live more sensibly. For instance we manage to persuade about one quarter of our cigarette smokers to either give up or reduce their smoking significantly. Similarly cholesterol levels can be brought down and early hypertension effectively treated. There are now good figures (see p. 52) showing the reduction in complications following long-term treatment of hypertension.

Breast cancer is the commonest cancer in women and the biggest single killer in middle age. If diagnosed early the survival rate is 85 per cent and, if left, this drops to 35 per cent, ie two-thirds of the cases are fatal. We now have good techniques for the detection of early disease and in our own clinic we find 7-8 new cases per 1000 women screened.

It is hoped that, as in America, health screening will increasingly be provided within industry and commerce and later spread to the so-called National Health Service, so that it can live up to its name and stop being what it is at present, namely a national sickness service.

Diagnosis apart, and this will be returned to in more detail shortly, the properly conducted health check has other advantages. It does provide a regular opportunity to sit down leisurely and review problems with a doctor. If all is well, reassurance, which is *not* a blank cheque for survival, is legitimate. If there are problems they can be dealt with.

The doctor can intervene, if necessary, in the relationship between the individual and his working environment. Acting as it were as the prisoner's friend, it is often possible to mitigate some of the conflicts and interpersonal clashes. The conditions under which this might be done are discussed later.

Wives like to know that their husbands are being looked after. Indeed we are frequently embarrassed by anxious wives, worried about their husbands, who expect us to be able to get their 'man' back into our clutches without letting him know where the motivation came from.

Additionally, husbands can discuss family problems and get advice about wives, children and relatives. They can also, and increasingly do, send their wives for a check-up too. About a fifth of the people we now see are women. It is surprising how often we can help on a family problem involving chronic illness. Executives tend not to see their family doctors unless they are 'ill'. They do not like to bother them about what they regard as trivia and also, particularly in London, going to the doctor means either missing work or bothering him on Saturday morning if he is there!

The health check then, which is done in working time, provides a diagnostic and environmental forum in which a wide variety of problems can be discussed and anxieties reviewed. As far as is humanly possible we try to achieve doctor-patient continuity and allocate one or two doctors to each company or executive group, so that there is a coherent overview. A 'patient's' first visit for a health check is primarily to chart his mental and physical baseline and to create his medical log book. Subsequent visits keep this up-to-date and record improvements and variations. In this way minor variations which may occur can be better evaluated against the general trend and background. Equally someone with, say, cardiograph abnormalities, falling into the hands of a new doctor, might be regarded as significantly diseased. The fact that these changes are known to have been present and unaltered for several years can be both a relief and reassurance. The medical

Factor	Per cent positive	Comment
HEREDITY Father died under 65 Mother died under 65	18.2 per cent 7.7 per cent	This puts about 1/3 in family risk group. About 40 per cent had 'coronary dead' fathers and mothers.
OBESITY	10 per cent or more o/wt 50 per cent 15 per cent o/wt 33.7 per cent 20 per cent o/wt 20.2 per cent	Half at some hazard: 1/5 seriously at risk
RAISED CHOLESTEROL	Moderately raised 30 per cent Seriously raised 9 per cent	40 per cent at hazard
RAISED BLOOD PRESSURE	Mild life insurance loading 30 per cent Serious loading 16 per cent	30 per cent loaded
SMOKING	0–20 cigarettes 16 per cent 20 plus 16 per cent Given up 31 per cent	One third at risk but another third have seen the light
CARDIOGRAPH ABNORMALITY	About 5 per cent definitly abnormal plus 4 per cent possibly abnormal	The Cardiograph can give early warning of heart damage

STRESS FACTORS

* A number of self employed taxi drivers come for regular checks

* Drive more than 20,000 mls. p.a.		14.0 per cent
Less than 2/52 holiday		9.4 per cent
More than 1 hrs. travel to work		10.4 per cent
Sleep problem	Recent	4.5 per cent
	Chronic	8.1 per cent
Feeling depressed		24.0 per cent
	Severe	4.7 per cent
	Suicidal thoughts	0.7 per cent
Life too demanding		11.6 per cent
Life not demanding enough		8.5 per cent
Personal money problems		16.8 per cent
Unhappy marriage		16.0 per cent
Nervous breakdown		
(Hospital or off work)		4.8 per cent

OTHER CONDITION

Liver damage – Alcohol	about	3.0 per cent
Reducing lung function – cigarettes	about	20.0 per cent
Possible diabetes		2.0 per cent

In addition, there were an appreciable number of hernias, haemorrhoids, varicose veins, mild anxiety states, etc.

Figure 14:1 Positive findings in coronary risk factors on 3000 men attending The Medical Centre for the first time in 1972. (Source: BUPA Medical Centre. Reprinted from *The Director*, June 1974) log book or long-term record is going to play an increasing role in guiding our thinking about the natural history of disease and the possible benefits of treatment. If computerized it lends itself to statistical analysis and easy recall.

The Medical Centre has now examined literally thousands of businessmen and we continue to be alarmed by the range of abnormalities that we find. Figure 14:1 is reprinted from an article in *The Director* of June 1974 and it lists the prevalence of a number of coronary risk factors in a group of 3000 men recently analysed by our research department. In addition, there is a steady yield of clinical conditions requiring treatment, like varicose veins, hernias, liver failure etc.

This is not the place to discuss these findings in detail, but they are included to substantiate the point that about a third of the people who come to The Medical Centre appear to be harbouring significant and unsuspected disease. If these figures are broken down into ten-year age groups, early changes are found at all ages. In the under 35's these are particularly alarming as they probably represent those most likely to succumb to a coronary 10-15 years later.

The principle of screening is that it is a method of identifying potentially vulnerable people and then doing further tests to confirm or deny this. I profoundly believe that this is the only possible way in which to reduce the appalling toll of coronary heart disease and we owe it to ourselves, our families and our firms to get these tests regularly carried out. Health maintenance is prudence not hypochondria.

Benefit to the firm

Individuals and the organization for which they work are, for better or worse, more or less married to each other. Although both partners use the marriage as a means to an end, they both should have a vested interest in the reasonable survival of the participants. If this is so, and it seems to be in well-conducted companies, firstly, the partners have a responsibility not to over exploit each other, or drive too hard a bargain, and secondly, the company at least must look after and protect its assets. The people who work for it are often the least replaceable of these assets and require looking after in at least the same way as other plant and machinery.

Coming back to the analogy of the motor car, the company who owns it should ensure regular maintenance and the executive who drives it should do so with reasonable care.

In addition, individuals and their wives like to feel that they are both cared about and looked after; this is particularly true of middle management who very much appreciate the provision of this type of health care. To offer, for instance, a periodic visit to a special women's screening unit to a loyal and long serving middle-aged woman can give an enormous lift to her morale.

A difficult area is always the extent to which an individual's anxieties and problems are, or should be, the concern of the company. This is a very difficult question to answer, but it is certain that should these press on the man, the anxiety will certainly reduce his effectiveness and the firm is inevitably concerned. In any case, in good firms, they want to help if they can, without being patronizing or paternal, and usually it is to the firm that the individual turns when he needs financial help or general advice. Thus it is convenient for the firm (as part of its asset protecting activity) to provide a means of doing this without getting directly involved in the man's personal or family affairs.

Similarly, an increasing number of companies provide, for similar reasons, BUPA or other sickness insurance cover, for exployees and their dependents. This is an accepted fringe benefit not currently taxable against the individual and allowable as a cost against the companies' revenue expenditure.

On a recent visit to America I was intrigued to meet a man who earned his living advising Trades Unions about the kind of fringe benefits they should negotiate with management and how these can be covered by insurance, etc. Periodic medical examinations were one of the items included in this package. The union then went on to quote this as a benefit of membership in its own competition for new members.

The New York Port Authority offers every one of its 20 000 employees the possibility of regular medical examinations, done in their own, now semi-automated, medical department. This was obviously of very great value. The American coverage, from the janitor to the president, cannot yet be provided over here, but most large organizations now provide executive health examinations and The Medical Centre provides schemes for over 500 companies of all sizes.

Benefit to the community

Progress is seldom made by governments or the 'establishment'. I hope that I have made out a case for the value of health maintenance. I have also implied that the concepts are not entirely accepted by older members of the medical profession, and one can only receive treatment or investigation from the NHS in relation to a complaint or symptom. Since industry creates the wealth on which the survival of our society depends, it is desirable that its managers, particularly, should be fit and effective as well as being at least as well looked after as its other assets.

In fact, in this area executives and their companies are setting a new trend and by pioneering the practice of health supervision, its general acceptance into the health/sickness service will be expedited.

It is very difficult to quantify the benefits of preventive medicine because the time base is extended, the statistics complicated and the follow-up of individual cases difficult, but Figure 14:2 shows some American figures in which an 'executively-examined' group were compared with the 'normal' lives in a life insurance company. In both groups, the 'treated' ie those examined, have appreciably lower mortality, thus illustrating the apparent benefit of regular examinations.

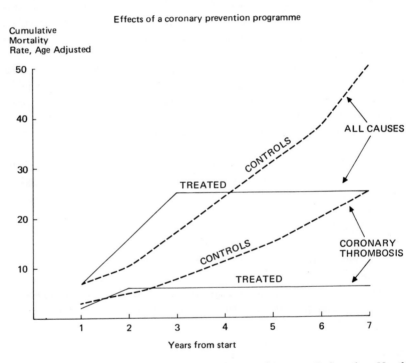

Figure 14:2 Benefits of screening programmes (Source: J. Stamler, North-West University, Chicago)

Over the years we have battled with doctors about the desirability of trying to deal with these problems and have been told that all we do is to turn people into anxious hyperchondriacs. In 1964 the treatment of hypertension was regarded as heresy, now the treatment of raised cholesterol is becoming accepted. Sadly there are still a few of what we call 'the come back when you are dead' type of doctor about, but they are a diminishing band. The public demand for preventive medicine has always been ahead of the medical professions' willingness to supply, but partly because medicine has to be consumer sensitive, priorities are happily changing.

The changing of priorities on which progress in any area depends is always a painful process for the vested interests involved. Practitioners of all professions, faced with the necessity for change have reluctantly to learn to do new and different things in perhaps an altered context. This is what is happening with preventive medicine and industry is playing its part in achieving this.

It is always said in this type of respect, that we cannot afford the cost of change either in terms of money or resources. Unfortunately in medicine sudden death is relatively cheap, especially if it occurs outside hospital, whereas prevention, which is an on-going activity, is inevitably more expensive. Thus academic medical economists and learned professors in their ivory towers currently have a happy time pontificating about the appalling cost of 'preventing' say a case of IHD or breast cancer. They proclaim, with the administrators and the vested interests, that this type of change is something we cannot conceivably afford. Most progress in any area is made over the dead body of the establishment, in our case the BMA, but with the encouragement of our 'customers' we are happy martyrs.

What should be done and who should do it?

In my view, executive health maintenance examinations should be regarded as an expert procedure and should only be done by doctors who are knowledgable about and interested in the way in which businessmen live and work.

The commonest routine medical examination is the life insurance medical in which doctor and 'prospectant' sit down and complete a usually largely misdirected questionnaire, before the former carries out a very simple physical examination based on a rough assessment of kidney function, blood pressure and weight. Doctors tend to regard this as relatively easy money and some, if asked to do executive examinations, treat these in much the same way.

There should be two distinct parts to the procedure. First the diagnostic profile in which a series of basic parameters are measured. Unlike the early American approach, the sky is not the limit as far as investigations are concerned. The object is not to do the maximum but the minimum number of investigations compatible with reasonable cost and the identification of early signs of disease.

It is not possible or sensible to look for early signs of all disease, such as cancer anywhere in the body, or test the brain for unsuspected epilepsy. It is only worth looking for relatively common conditions like IHD and possibly lung and prostatic cancer. A common extravagance, in my view, is the routine use of intestinal x-rays — the Barium meal. In the USA these used to be done routinely, as did special rectal examinations involving the passage of an instrument to examine the inside of the lower colon. Barium meals are expensive, mildly time consuming and involve a moderate amount of radiation exposure. In the absence of digestive symptoms they seldom reveal unexpected disease, except possibly in Japanese in whom stomach cancer is common.

There is no need for the subject to be incarcerated in a hospital or nursing home and the investigations should be done within a couple of hours. Currently, apart from recording personal, occupational and medical details we do the following investigations:

1   Accurate measurement of height and weight.
2   Lung function.
3   Recording of blood pressure and electrocardiograph.
4   Hearing and vision testing to make sure that there is no need for expert assessment regarding glasses or hearing aid.
5   Full size chest and abdominal x-rays.
6   Simple urine test, backed by a more detailed one if the former reveals abnormality.
7   Blood sample for biochemical and haematological examination.

The biochemical profile is probably the most important single investigation and its content varies with changing technology and the introduction of more precise tests. Abnormality in one of the first line tests, like raised blood sugar indicating the possibility of diabetes, should lead more or less automatically to second line tests which proceed to a more precise diagnosis. But there is no point in doing the second line tests unless a specific need for them is indicated.

Patients going to hospitals and doctors' surgeries have been conditioned by the inefficiency of the system to be endlessly patient and to wait quietly in queues and trail from department to department for x-rays, blood tests and so on. Busy businessmen coming for a routine check should not accept this approach, any more than they would take their expensive car to a badly organized garage. Their health check investigations should be done expeditiously in one place, in one dressing gown and under the umbrella of a single appointment. This implies a specialized unit rather than the traditional clinically orientated hospital.

The second item is the consultation with a doctor. If I have not made it clear that, in my view, this should be psychosomatically orientated, I have failed in the purpose of this book. A simple 'laying on of clinical hands', as in life insurance examinations, is inadequate.

There should be a detailed and leisurely interview aimed at discovering what problems the individual has and how he is dealing with them. Problems should be looked for in the areas of work, home and leisure. If there are problems, symptoms or overt illness then further questions should be asked: *why* is he ill? as well as *what* is wrong with him? All this takes time and inevitably puts up the cost, because expert time is money. At least an hour should be available for each interview and as said previously, the doctor must be interested and experienced enough to talk intelligently about the work situation.

As well as this, there should be a simple physical examination followed by a counselling session in which the results and findings are discussed and advice given. Some people like to do this at a second visit, but this is extravagant in time, and at a well-run centre most of the results should be available to the doctor when the patient is seen. Any properly oriented doctor *can* do this work, but rather few of them have the interest and general practitioners seldom the time. The choice lies between the personal family doctor, the company doctor, if there is one, a nominated consultant or a special unit such as The Medical Centre.

The individual wants good and disinterested advice about himself. As his problems may be highly personal or involve his relationships at work, it could be, especially if he is a senior person, that both the company doctor and his GP are too close to him. It is usually wise to avoid close, personal relationships with one's advisers like doctors and lawyers. The man you play golf or drink sherry with may not be the best person to get involved over family anxieties or personal misdemeanors. Equally, the company doctor who has an administrative relationship with the general manager or personnel director may be well advised to keep clear of their family or personal problems. Involvement in a difficult situation would inevitably feed back into his administrative relationship. Again the man you have lunch with is not necessarily the man you want to talk to about yourself.

The company, who mostly pay for the examinations, have a number of options as to what they think is in it for them. These will be outlined subsequently but they ought to make sure that the examination is competently and expertly done and this means that they should nominate the doctor or doctors available and not leave it to the individual choice of their executives. One of the benefits of the procedure is to get an overview of the executive group and not to have them seen entirely as individuals. This again means that one or two doctors should do all the company's examinations. To allow each man to go to a doctor of his own choice, and to finish up with as many standards and views as there are executives, does not seem to be the way to get value for what is after all considerable expenditure.

Two other compromises are possible. The first, which is very convenient and productive, is for the doctor on the medical centre to work through the company doctor. With, as always, the patient's permission, a detailed report is sent to him as it is to the GP. Depending on his relationship with the company and the executive, it is then up to him to decide what use is made of the information. It allows him, perhaps while personally seeing more junior staff, to know what is going on without getting deeply involved. In other cases the industrial medical officer organizes and monitors the service, but neither he nor the company require a report.

The second and growing possibility is for medical centres to use their specialized expertise and equipment to generate the diagnostic profile which then goes to the industrial medical officer or outside doctor who conducts the consultation. This works well provided he is properly orientated. In fact The Medical Centre was set up partly to provide this facility for general practitioners and to encourage them to do preventive medicine.

In summary, the examination consists of two parts: diagnostic profile and clinical counselling session. Both are expert procedures and should be done by an interested and experienced doctor who does at least enough of this type of work to give sensible answers, as well as medical advice.

Using the information

The most vexed question about executive health examinations is the problem of what, if any, information about the individual goes back to the company and, if so, to whom it should go. Before discussing this let us deal first with the easier aspects of reporting.

The most important person is the individual concerned, and surely he has a right to know about himself. The man should be given as much information as he can digest and understand. It is explained to him what has gone wrong and what the problems and possibilities are. Experience has shown that this approach promotes the best motivation in altering life styles or taking long-term medication, etc.

The next step is to ask the man's permission to send a medically detailed report to his own doctor for his records and so that he can discuss, initiate and supervise any treatment or further investigations. It must be realized that an executive health examination is advisory only and that no treatment can be given. Being devoted to preventive medicine at The Medical Centre, we may advise treatment which some doctors regard as meddlesome or unnecessary, but we are entitled to our view and equally the GP is entitled to disagree with it. Should this happen the patient will have to discuss it with the GP and if necessary decide whose advice he is going to take. As in management, there can be more than one answer to a problem and doctors should not be so childish as to feel that they cannot be disagreed with or to expect to play God all the time.

Should the man have no doctor or have no confidence in the one with whom he is nominally registered, but need treatment or supervision, he will expect advice about how to get into contact with a doctor with whom he is in sympathy. If there is no need for treatment or supervision the records can be kept in The Medical Centre *pro tem.*

Executives who travel a lot and who have medical problems, or are on long-term drugs, may be well advised to carry a detailed medical report about with them in case it is needed in foreign countries. In fact being ill away from home is both hazardous and expensive. If at all possible it is wise to fly home, and there are few diseases that will not stand this. Otherwise one needs good local advice and additional sickness insurance cover as provided by BUPA Worldwide Travel and other similar policies.

Who in the company?

Reporting back to the company can range from no reports at all to full and detailed ones being sent by the doctor without any reference to the individual, who does not know what has been said. At The Medical Centre, if it can possibly be avoided, we will not operate under the latter code. We feel that it is better for the company to have some report and either be reassured that all is well or participate in dealing with any problem. We also feel very strongly that no information should be disclosed without the express permission of the individual, who should also be told, at least in outline, what is going to be said. If there is a medical or behavioural problem which either arises from or affects the work situation, it can only be dealt with by reference to the company and in relation to the options reasonably available. On the whole, management can only be helpful if it knows what the problem is and what the details are. To expect full management cooperation but to withold all medical details is to ask for an unreasonably blank cheque. As already mentioned, employer and employee have mutual interests which are best served by having confidence in each other.

Increasingly now this confidence exists and with growing participation in each others affairs, the value of free exchange of information about individuals is being more and more accepted. If an individual has personal or family problems the company does not need or want to get involved, it only wants to facilitate their solution. But otherwise it helps best by knowing what the problem is. At The Medical Centre we like to have the right, always with the man's permission, to report to and discuss medical reports with a nominated senior person in the company, for example the chairman.

Much anxiety is generated by the suspicion that medical information may ruin or hold up an individual's career and restrict promotion. Perhaps it will, but should a company be expected to promote an unfit person who cannot stand the strain and who might well let down both himself and the company by getting, say, a coronary? This is a very difficult problem area and it is imperative that the medical situation is taken into account when considering people for key appointments, and that management should be entitled to ask for this advice.

Doctors should not want to play God and become king makers, and they need to get used to their advice not necessarily being taken all the time, but they should be willing to give it and their patients should be willing for it to be given. After all, the object of the exercise is to try to make the best deal or compromise for both parties. The individual seldom suffers from this interchange and in the great majority of cases the doctor can play a useful role in redeploying or reducing tension and pressure.

Another interesting and useful area of this type of work, is the general discussion with the chairman about the climate within his organization and how it compares with others. If I, or one of my staff, have seen twenty or so executives from a company, not only have we advised and assessed them personally, we must also have formed opinions about the group and the organization as a whole. In this context one can discuss climates and behaviour patterns without, if necessary, mentioning any names.

Chairmen find this dialogue very useful and we do not hesitate to criticize the chairman if this seems justified. Being independant, one can tell him the home truths about himself which his colleagues have not been brave enough to mention. By so doing, sometimes one can dramatically improve the climate within the organization.

I am strongly in favour of this type of relationship and, while accepting that there may be situations when no reporting is the best solution, it still seems that in these cases the most value is not being had from the procedures.

The examinations are best instigated on a voluntary basis and no attempt should be made to make them obligatory for existing staff. They can later become a condition of service within the company. It is often helpful if the chairman, or whoever is to be responsible, comes first as a guinea pig. He can then write to his colleagues and say that he has personally been through the mill. The precise needs of a company vary and it is useful to discuss the terms of reference for a scheme in the right of the guinea pig examination. The terms should then be fully set out and agreed by the individuals. It is essential that each individual should know what he is in for and what is involved before he comes. To minimize misunderstanding we ask for a signed permission to report.

Any doctoring unit can only be helpful if it has the full confidence of the individual and he feels that the unit is primarily there to help him. At The Medical Centre if we feel that a man is overstretched and harrassed, and we would only do this if we were on strong ground, we will make it our business to convince him that his work situation needs discussing. Usually the man knows and subconsciously realizes that he has his back to the wall and mostly our intervention is received with gratitude. If, however, permission is refused there is no more that we can do.

It is also worth emphasizing the point that negative reports are as valuable and more encouraging than adverse ones. Individuals and companies benefit from being told that the troops are in good heart and standing up well.

Special examinations

A different area of discussion comes from situations like the pre-employment medical examination or the 'problem reference' situation. In the former, a company is entitled to a detailed report about a new employee in whom money will be invested in training, and on whom the future of the enterprise may well rest. To take on such a man without a medical is like buying a house without a survey, or a secondhand car without looking under the bonnet. It is folly. But here too we would want the individual to know what we said so that, if the report is adverse, at least he can get something done about the problem. A lot of executives have been helped in this way.

Individuals do have breakdowns, get illnesses which affect their work capacity, or just become less effective. It may be that the man will have to be demoted or retired, but before deciding what is best for both of them, an expert medical report, in relation to work capacity, is essential. Here again the company is entitled to a confidential report and the individual is stupid if he either resents the suggestion or refuses the examination.

Another area of great interest is to be asked either 'am I' or 'is this man' standing up well to great strain? Or again, 'am I' or 'is he' doing too much and being dangerously overloaded? There is obviously no dogmatic answer to this question, one can only express a quality judgement, but the better one knows the man and his company the more accurate the opinion is likely to be. This is a further argument in favour of continuity of executive health supervision and the facility to be able to interpret the present in relation to previous baseline measurements.

Organization of examinations

The following are a few last points of detail about the organization of executive health examinations.

How often should they be done?

As yet, there is no statistical answer to this problem Our advice is as follows:

Age 50 and over — annually
40-50 — every two years
Under 40 — every three years

But one needs to keep the guidelines flexible; senior people, harassed people, travellers and those with problems may need to be seen more often. We like to say that when they have all been seen once, we will tell you when we want to see them again. Usually, on average and for budget purposes, it works out at about every eighteen months.

Who should be included?

This is much more difficult because organizations are hierarchial and there must be cut-off points in relation to salary and status. One does not want the examination to be a status symbol *per se,* but this is difficult to avoid. The important thing is to include the bright youngsters on the way up, even if they are not seen very often. It is useful for them to know that a helping hand is available, and often they do get stressed by over-promotion and sudden executive responsibility.

Usually in deciding where to stop one comes to rest in middle management, the £5-£6000 a year salary bracket, but in smaller organizations there may be key people earning less than this who ought to be included.

Staff going overseas and those who travel a lot should probably be seen annually. If at all possible women should be included and senior secretaries and other loyal servants very much appreciate being sent to a special women's screening unit, for instance. Opinions differ about whether companies should pay for wives to come and this usually becomes rather expensive. In morale terms it is obviously likely to be a good thing and very much appreciated but, as yet, few companies have found this a justifiable expenditure.

Husbands and wives like the idea that both are being looked after and I suspect that companies will increasingly be willing to pay some of the cost. A growing number of husbands certainly do.

How much should be done?

As has been said, we like to do the minimum necessary to detect common diseases and to be able to ask for additional examinations or second line tests, when these are clinically indicated. As they are medically indicated, second line tests can be claimed against BUPA or other sickness insurance policies. The examination itself cannot be claimed, as there is no insurance element, but BUPA does have rebate schemes for its group subscribers attending The Medical Centre.

Tax situation

Under the present regulations a medical examination, paid for by the company and done at their request is not taxable, as a benefit in kind to the individual. This is reinforced if the company gets even the most general report to the effect that the examination has been carried out and the man is fit or recommended to receive treatment. Similarly BUPA and similar benefits paid for by the company are expense tax deductable.

FIFTEEN

Checklist for retirement

My aim, as a preventively oriented doctor, is to keep people fit and lively in the hope that ultimately they will die quickly and suddenly in ripe old age. To maximize the chances of this happening, retirement needs to be given as much thought and priority as the other major phases of life. Health in retirement is governed by exactly the same rules as health at all other times. Thus, the mental approach to, and the reduction of stress, in retirement, is just as important as it is earlier in life. Perhaps even more so, because as horizons narrow, range of choice is essential.

At the Institute of Directors, we have also tried to help our retiring members through the Retirement Advisory Bureau, established over ten years ago. This now has a wealth of experience and contacts to advise members about retirement activity. Its main object is to put social and other organizations in touch with men looking for largely voluntary work and to advise individuals as to the sort of opportunities which might be available in their area. Experience here has shown that three years is not too far ahead to start making suitable arrangements.

Retirement presents two entirely different sets of problems. The first concerns the currently extremely unsatisfactory attitude of the community towards its retired members. The second concerns the individual and his own attitudes and problems. As it is misunderstood and neglected, the first area is worth brief mention, particularly since it provides the background against which the individual must operate.

Retirement and the community

In our society, we label and judge people by what they do. One's status and identity is established by what one does: stockbroker, businessman, doctor, rodent executive, etc. The fact that we now tend to invent and accept high status sounding names for the essential but more humble jobs does not make the situation any easier when the man retires.

However, once people retire they lose their status and identity and tend to become 'non-people' in their own eyes and the eyes of others. There is little exciting about a retired civil servant who might have been anything from a permanent secretary to a post office clerk. In addition, we make it almost impossible for retired people to remain integrated in the community. They get something called an old age pension. They are then additionally clobbered with the earnings rule, which actively discourages them from contributing gainful work to the community, which often desperately needs what they can or could do, particularly in a service capacity. Doing things for other people, even if it is serving in a shop, replaces the social contact which is an essential part of work.

For a variety of reasons too, we seem to allow large congregations of retired 'non-people' to collect in allegedly salubrious areas and form a sort of 'costa geriatrica'. We neither venerate nor look after our aged and in a variety of ways we make their lives as difficult rather than as easy as we can. By 1980 which, politicians permitting, is not all that far off, there will be well over ten million people, about a fifth of the population, in the retirement group. This is too large a slice of the community to have 'out on a limb'. These numbers, too may well be swollen by the increasing tendency towards earlier rather than later retirement.

Another frightening thing about this situation is that it means that about a third of the population is being educated, a third working and a third retired, ie at any one time only about one third is working really productively. It could be that this as a luxury we should not afford. It is sometimes thought that this situation has occurred because people are living longer. In fact, this is not the substantial case. Average life expectancy has only gone up two or three years in the last twenty-five, but because of improvements in standards of living and medical care, far more people are surviving into retirement.

If a man achieves the age of 65 in reasonably good health, the statistics say, he can expect to live more than ten years. This does not contradict the earlier statement on life expectancy, which is an inevitably overall average, based on expectancy from childhood or early adult life. Another factor which we have to consider in this respect is the special problem of women, because so many of them outlive their husbands and become the lonely elderly.

As already mentioned, a proportion of them will already be widows by the time their husbands would normally expect to retire. Most of the rest of them will die as widows because women of all ages live longer than men. For reasons which we do not understand, and which are far from obvious, women are far tougher than men. This finally becomes a disadvantage because on the whole men die suddenly and women tend to linger and become bedridden, but this is a problem outside our present scope. Thus, provision for retirement also involves some hard and straight thinking about what is going to happen to the woman when her husband dies.

Businessmen tend to make very bad retirement material. One of their diseases, and another one not included in text books of medicine, is the 'it can't happen to me syndrome', paraphrased as 'delusions of indestructability'. Things happen to others, *they* have problems, but I am all right, is what this type of man says to himself. His wife is too frightened of him to point out how much at hazard he might be or how worried she is about him. For reasons which we have already fully explored, there is a horrible tendency for our businessman to suddenly arrive at retirement without having done nearly enough contingency planning. A feature of this species of *Home Sapiens* is to resist thinking about himself until it is too late. Thus, if he survives without getting a coronary, he may well suddenly find himself clutching his gold clock, the last thing he now wants, and wending his lonely way home with nothing much to do tomorrow.

He suddenly realizes that he has no office to go to, no train to catch, no secretary to organize him, nothing in the diary. He has neither status nor identity, and unless he has been clever and sensible, he has nothing to do, which can be awful after the first few mornings of lying in late and days of extra golf. This man will become miserable, behave like a bear with a sore head, fall out with his wife, who is not used either to having her house occupied or providing lunch seven days a week, and may well drift into a disillusioned and resentful depression.

A group who experience extra hazards in retirement are those who have spent most or all of their lives with a single, self-centred and inward looking organization. Employees get indoctrinated with the concept of how lucky they are to be part of such a solicitous and all-caring fraternity. Work, leisure, social activity and a number of economic perks are all company centred. This living, working, and thinking about and for a company may be splendid from the company's point of view, to provide it with devoted servants, but is dangerous for the individual who loses touch with the real outside world. When he is suddenly faced with retirement he is sucked dry, insecure and rather lonely without the support of his 'welfare nest'. The normal 'bereavement' is deeper than with ordinary retirement because one may really have to start all over again, and it could almost be too late. In my experience this over-involvement with the work group can provide retirement situations which are very difficult to adjust to. This is the type of man who may well fizzle out or drift melancholically down hill, to die within a year or two of a broken heart.

In the Pre-Retirement Association recently, we have been trying to help one or two organizations of this type to broaden their retirement base by running advisory courses for retirees. It appears that management now increasingly realises that it should at least provide the opportunity for its staff at all levels to prepare for retirement. Its continuing responsibility can be seen to be greater than the provision of a pension. Indeed a growing number are cooperating in the provision of part-time work activities centres., welfare schemes for old employees and so on. Preferably these should be more community based, but it is often easier for a large company to set them up. Retired people are desperate for activity and association. They want to go on belonging to something. One company runs its own switchboard very successfully with part-time pensioners.

Problems of redundancy

Before we look at the problems of retirement in a little more detail, it is worth looking briefly at the not dis-similar problems of redundancy and early retirement — voluntary or imposed. For a variety of reasons outside the scope of this book, an increasing number of businessmen have found or are finding themselves pushed out well before sixty. There is no longer room for them in what they were doing. Of course, this is a frightening and difficult situation. It is also one which is much easier to preach about than to solve. The first thing that happens is that the man's morale and self-esteem are totally destroyed. He either gets depressed or resentful or both. The world has treated him badly and probably owes him a living. This may well be true, but because of what his attitude does to him, he loads the dice against getting another job because the chips can be heard rattling on his shoulder.

To become saleable, this man has to try to sort out his attitude to an adversity, which may well mean reorganizing all his priorities. The best thing to do, even if he cannot afford it, is to go away for a holiday and try to recover from the shock. The next thing is to admit to all and sundry that this has happened, proclaim the need for help and put himself on the market. There are numerous stories of the redundant executive who will not admit it, even to his wife, and who goes on 'going to work' at least as long as the season ticket lasts, or until the redundancy pay runs out. Similarly, there are stories of retired people who go and watch their old work mates clock in and out of the factory or look lonely out of the window, counting the bricks on the wall opposite.

The redundant man has got to start off by dealing with his pride and then redeploy himself almost certainly at a lower level. He has got to be prepared to start again in almost any role, and then justify himself. The recently retired executive can be very like this, if he has not done his homework on retirement. The contingency planning should be aimed at avoiding loneliness in old age. This is what retirement planning is all about and it is seldom properly done. The one considerable advantage arising from retirement at 60 rather than 65 is that it should be easier to find things to do that will carry on for a few years when one is 60. The younger man is appreciably more employable perhaps on a part-time basis.

Planning

Several years before retirement, a man and his wife should have begun to find solutions to the following groups of problems. (They are described in greater detail in a book edited by Michael Pilch and sponsored by the Pre-Retirement Association called *The Retirement Book.*) These are well worth outlining here, if satisfactory answers are not available, the couple will be seriously dis-eased. Not only this, they will also fail to get the just reward for all the hard work which they have done. Ordered tranquillity is what is required in retirement and like everything else this has to be actively contrived.

The problem areas are as follows:

1 Activity
2 Finance
3 Residence
4 Health—mental and physical

Activity

'But uglier yet is the hump we get from having too little to do'. Kipling.

Work does more than just bring home the bacon. It gives, as we have just seen, status and identity; it also gives a sense of purpose and companionship, the importance of which is only realized when it is no longer available. Professor H.A. Jones of Leicester has called this work-place association 'distanced intimacy'. By this, he means that one can have a greater or lesser degree of contact without the obligations of social or family relations. The relationships are not demanding, but it is very comforting to be surrounded by people one knows

One of the major priorities on planning activity in retirement is to replace the distanced intimacy of work.

One of my private dreams is that before too long we shall set up a network of activities centres across the country. Run on a non-profit making basis, they would provide a focus where individuals could go and do things; and householders, organizations, companies, etc, could commission work of any and every simple sort. Most of us are frustrated carpenters. The work would be paid for as would the labourer. All it wants is imagination and acceptance by the unions who, incidentally, strangled our first attempt to do this.

Businessmen it was suggested, are likely to start off by being bad at retirement, because so many of them have confined their contacts to business associates and their other activities to trade and professional organizations. Sensible people should enter retirement with a quiver full of potential activities and usable contacts; it does not matter what they are, provided they are congenial.

Activities can be paid or unpaid, work related, or socially useful, cultural or 'enthusiastic', ie collecting and making things. Hopefully enough has been said to make the point that what is to be done needs both thinking about and planning for. It could, for instance, be worth considering evening classes to acquire new skills and interests to deploy on retirement. It is in this area that work for local voluntary associations becomes so valuable, they need your skill and you now have the time.

Some of the activity should be physical to get one out of doors, some should involve the wife as well, but please do not sit on the same committees. Another important factor is to find things, particularly as one gets older, that inevitably bring contact with other people. Being wanted and being able to help is of major importance, and in every community there is a need for voluntary help. There are a number of agencies and organizations that help to match the supply and demand of voluntary work. The Pre-Retirement Association can provide details about these.

There is another area that needs rethinking and this is the wife's activities. Her 'retirement' tends to start earlier than her husband's perhaps when the children leave home. By the time her husband retires she should be thoroughly organized and it is important that his coming home does not upset her activities. Having to get his lunch is no excuse. Make him get his own and make him responsible for some of the household chores. It all helps to fill the day and being regularly responsible is also a useful aim.

Being reasonably busy in a not too demanding way is the key to contentment in retirement and it will lead to good mental and bodily health. If the husband is well organized, the wife is likely to be contented too. If he is idling round under her feet, there is likely to be friction. On her part, she must realize that the home is now in constant use and she must expect father to tramp in from the garden looking for a cup of coffee.

Finance

We started our company-based retirement advisory seminars in a large organization which prides itself on its welfare state and pension coverage. We were able to demonstrate to them that many of their staff would welcome outside independent advice. In most pension schemes, for instance, there is a lump-sum option and dealing with this presents problems. We then moved on to a large central bank and, greatly daring, presumed to try to advise the managers themselves. We managed to make the point that there was a need for advice from outside experts in this particular field.

The upshot of this is that a lot of business men, perhaps in accordance with their general inability to look after their own affairs, can benefit considerably from expert advice on the organization of their resources as they enter retirement. In fact, financial planning is often the earliest priority, needing perhaps ten years to really get it right.

In addition, there is a need to learn about social security regulations, the earnings rule and so on. The main problem is in finding out what you have got, deciding what to do, for instance, do you need or want to leave money to your children? What provision to make for your widow? This is very important because firstly, it is highly likely that there will be a widow to be provided for, and secondly, residual pensions for widows tend to be inadequate under most schemes. Another point here, and this may be part of the great unwillingness to discuss death and dying, is the question of whether your wife fully understands what to do and where she stands, should anything happen to you. It is important to know where your will is, who the executors are, how much money will she have, and so on.

A further point worth rethinking is the value of the house. For many people apart from their pensions the house is their only or main asset. Its mortgage is likely to have been paid and there will now be a case for recapitalizing it in some way so that you, rather than your heirs, have the use of the money. For instance, is it really necessary to leave money to your children who are often doing better than you did at their age?

A financial expert could provide a useful checklist for you in relation to your responsibilities and resources. He could also advise about the best ways of hedging against inflation, the case for annuities ans so on. It is now our very considerable experience that although money is often the least important aspect of retirement, many people could get a better return on whatever they have by better advice. The statement that money is the least important aspect may sound surprising, but it is as true as any generalization ever is.

We seldom have enough money at any time, or would always like more. Come retirement you have to make the best of what you have got even if this means going out to work part-time. However, in practice, and with a lot of skill, people can and do exist on the state pension plus, if necessary, supplementary benefit. In practice money turns out to be less of a problem than activity and attitude of mind, which largely conditions health.

Residence

The concept of the retirement bungalow on the hill above the sea, or the flat on the 'costa somewhere or other', needs very careful thought. The seaside can be pretty foul in winter and the hill tough to carry the shopping up ten years later. People who put their money into, say, Malta, ten years ago, are feeling pretty insecure now. To push the problem to the extreme, take the case of the couple who retire, lose their status and identity, sell their house and retreat to Eastbourne, for example. They arrive, know nobody, have little to do and rapidly become depressed and lonely 'non-people'. It is worse in the wilds of the country, and far worse still in small expatriate groups living in the sun on foreign soil and talking to each other about the old days.

As emphasized all along, the most important single thing in retirement for most people, is activity and social contact. Thus, one should aim at the maximum involvement potential, so as to maintain contacts late into life. For all sorts of reasons, this is far more likely to occur in the area one has lived most of one's life than it is in a new area one comes to as an elderly stranger. For these and many other reasons, remaining in the same place or very near it, is strongly recommended.

A further and important point about moving is that, on the whole, women find it more difficult than men, particularly as they get older, to grow new roots and make new social contacts. Moving can be disastrous to a slightly shy over middle-aged woman. If there are good reasons for moving, and there may well be, it is wise to try and do this well ahead of retirement, so that new local identity can be established beforehand. Thus, the second home, if it exists, can become the retirement home. A last point here is that the so called retirement areas which make up the 'costa geriatrica' need to be avoided, because they are too full of retired people looking backwards. The population is out of balance and the social services increasingly inadequate to deal with the demands.

Having decided where to live, the next step is what to live in, size of house, size of garden, room for grandchildren and family and so on. For instance, a colleague of mine advises against any garden bigger than his wife can manage. It is likely that the house you have lived in all your life is unlikely to be a convenient house to retire or die in. Inevitably age ultimately brings frailty and diminished physical resources. Something like a nice warm bungalow, or flat in a block with a lift, is likely to be better than a Victorian-type house with stairs. Taking the final view, it is wise to provide something that one person can manage alone unless it is known that there is a friendly family waiting.

Health

Very little more need be said about this, because the ground has already been fully covered but two points do need emphasis. The first is that the best laid plans and involvements will be vitiated by the wrong mental approach.

Most people, given the choice, would like to go on working at a reduced rate more or less until they drop, but there are a lot of good reasons why this cannot be. Unless one is professionally engaged or running one's own organization, provision must be made for the needs of the other younger people in the team.New ideas and winds of change should be allowed for. The other point here is that, idealistic though it may sound, having done one kind of activity for forty odd years, surely the time is ripe to be brave and enjoy a different way of life with new and less demanding priorities.

This is what we hope retirement is all about, the final reward for the routine effort of work should be the relative freedom to enjoy frenzied tranquility in a way you and your wife like. Achieving something along these lines will make for high morale and new challenges. Entering retirement resenting everything, and feeling that the world owes you yet another break, is a prescription for depression and possibly an early death. At the least it will provoke dis-ease: recreation is similarly re-creation.

The second point is to realize that the investment, wise or unwise, that you have previously made in health, will now, hopefully, pay a good dividend. However, lungs worn out by forty years of filter tips will cough their way to early breathlessness, unused joints will creak, flabby muscles rebel and so on. It is essential to get into good order before retirement and even more important to regard the maintenance as a vital discipline as you get older.

Sensible diet, weight control, ruthless pursuit of exercise summer and winter, regular medical checks, attention to hearing and vision, etc, helps towards comfort. 'Wall in for winter' but have plenty to do and still get out regularly.

As age advances, some disabilities will be inevitable. Do not be proud about them. Use a stout stick on slippery days. Be careful about accident hazards in the house and so on. In retirement there is no reason for not looking after and cosseting oneself. Minor conditions should be treated with more respect. Stay in for a cold and have a couple of days in bed, if at all necessary. Regular winter 'flu injections are strongly advocated. Chronic chests should also have regular winter antibiotic cover. Ask your doctor about these.

Lastly, lucky is the man or woman who finishes life without the need for doctors and medical services. It is desirable to make satisfactory medical arrangements, and these could be a factor in finally deciding where to live, ie an area remote from hospital or nursing home is likely to be under-doctored. It is often not easy to find a doctor who is conscientious about his older patients and group practices may be efficient but a bit impersonal, especially for the elderly, who want personal service. It is prudent to shop around and try to find a suitable doctor in practice. The first choice will have to be whether to rely on the NHS or perhaps remain as a private patient. Most businessmen will have had some sort of sickness insurance cover during their working life. There is a tendency now for the more enlightened organizations to keep this going as a retirement perk. If not, it may be difficult to afford, but there is a lot to be said for trying to continue what you have been used to. Often the private patient has a wider choice than in the health service.

Whatever the decision, it is essential to make contact with your doctor, get to know him, see that he knows all about you, so that when something does go wrong, he has the essential information about the family. Hopefully the doctor you choose will be sensible enough to provide a maintenance service for his older patients. Remember too, that medicine is a consumer service so do not be frightened of demanding what is your just due. After all, it is paid for out of taxes.

The last area that needs re-emphasis is that of family relationships. They are now, with narrowing horizons, more vital than they have ever been before. Retirement can be like getting married all over again. Couples are likely to be embarking on a seven day week together. This will need a lot of thought and readjustment. If the previous relationship was not particularly good a few fences will have to be mended. If it was rather bad and survived because of the separation, closer proximity may well produce misery and all kinds of aches and pains.

The domestic situation must be discussed, assessed and new priorities allocated with friendly frankness. This is one of the reasons why we think that planning for retirement is just as important as the other areas of education and learning. Because the economic options are almost non-existent and activity requires very high motivation, successful retirement is that last great test of character and ability.

Index